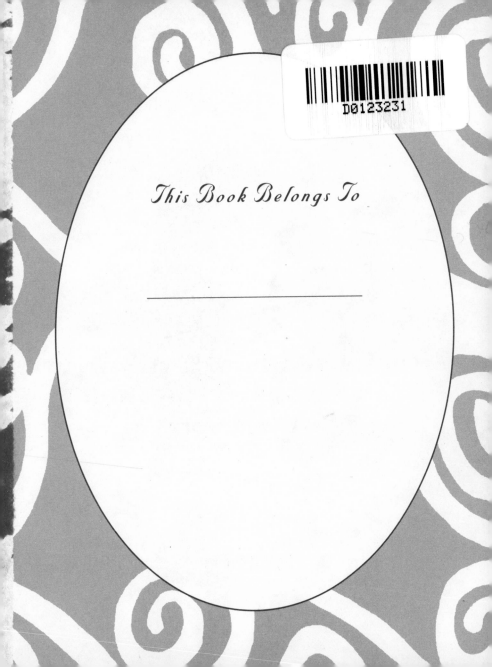

This Book Belongs To

_____

Monique Jellerette deJongh & Cassandra Marshall Cato-Louis

NEW YORK LONDON TORONTO SYDNEY AUCKLAND

HOW TO MARRY A BLACK MAN

The Real Deal

PUBLISHED BY DOUBLEDAY
a division of Bantam Doubleday Dell Publishing Group, Inc.
1540 Broadway, New York, New York 10036

DOUBLEDAY and the portrayal of an anchor with a dolphin are
trademarks of Doubleday, a division of Bantam Doubleday Dell
Publishing Group, Inc.

Illustrations by Barbara Brandon
Designed by Bonni Leon-Berman
Hieroglyphs by Anthony E. Blow

Excerpt from *Healing Pluto Problems* (York Beach, Maine: Samual Weiser, 1986)
on page 63, 64 is used by permission.

Library of Congress Cataloging-in-Publication Data
Applied For
ISBN 0-385-48246-9

Printed in the United States of America
February 1996
1   3   5   7   9   10   8   6   4   2
First Edition

Bobby, I adore you . . .

Your being able to put up with me

convinces me never to underestimate you again.

How do you keep making me fall in love with you?

MoJ

I lovingly dedicate this book to my husband

Elmer "Papi" Supriano Louis,

who saved my life and gave me gifts of love

that I will cherish eternally.

C.

Thanks to friends who always knew . . .

janet

marie

bobby de

elmer

paul

dylan

jordan

layla

desiree

tar

moshood

z

barbara b

dr. rich h.

dr. rocchio

emma & the team at d

carole anne/gj

grace

pat

patty

taylor, bernadette & scott

hattie

al/papa aj

alvin

ann carol

mike carroll

ingrid & sigfried

sandra & the people at
 Servisio Kultura in

Curaçao, Netherlands
 Antilles

alda jr.

linda, ariel, erica & darrel

fire marshal grandma and
 grandpa al

vaughan & nikki

danielle, taylor, troy &
 diane

nana, gramamma, grand gg,
 grandaddy, aunt rita, criso,
 bob & momma donna

renee, linda r, alexandra,
 nicole teru & beth +1

ayka, katsue & doug

freddie & beve

giselle & desiree—queens-
 borough public library

claude e

sean

all the men who weren't
 The Ones but who
 helped us to know who
 he was when we met him

all the men who partici-
 pated in the focus
 groups/interviews

all the womben who par-
 ticipated in the focus

groups/sistah to sistah
 conversations

danielle

moutique, olu o'risha &
 ade

linda

tony

lynda & jim

sierra

craig & tommy

lisa

michael

clyde

chase, chelsea, chet, char-
 lene & bart

sandra, justin, evan & iris

alex, aisha, angela & taylor

aqueelah & margie

arnela

sonja

paula

sarita & dan

jules & jeff

robin

chris & beverly

amtrak & employees

wendy

arletta & rudy

dad & liz

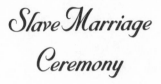

Slave Marriage Ceremony

Dark an stormy may come de wedder;

I jines dis he-male an' dis she-male togedder.

Let none, but Him dat makes de thunder,

Put dis he-male an' dis she-male asunder.

I darfore 'nounce you bofe de same.

Be good, go 'long, an' keep up yo' name.

De broomstick's jumped, de world's not wide.

She's now yo' own. Salute yo' bride!

From: *Crossing the Danger Water*
Three Hundred Years of African-American Writing

CoNTENTS

Phase II
Gettin' a Brothah to Notice the New You

Phase III
Reality Check

Mo' Stuff

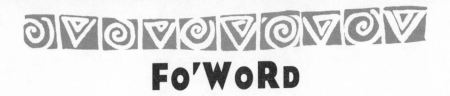

Fo'WoRd

WE DARE YOU . . .

. . . to face the biggest obstacle that is keeping you from getting married to a Black man: *you!* Go stand in front of the mirror. Look deeply into your own eyes and answer these questions silently to yourself:

Do I want to get married?	**Y N**
Am I ready to get married?	**Y N**
Although I'm powerful, do I believe that I will find a Black man that can deal with me?	**Y N**
Do I believe that there are Black men out there who aren't in jail, taken, or gay?	**Y N**
Do I really believe that there is someone out there for me?	**Y N**
Am I ready to change the way I've been going about flirting with Black men?	**Y N**
Am I ready to get serious about taking someone else's life into my hands?	**Y N**

Can I love someone else as much as I love myself? **Y N**

Am I ready to have sex with only one person for the rest of
my life? **Y N**

Have I healed all of my past heartaches to allow my husband in? **Y N**

If you answered "Yes" to most of these questions, then get prepared to walk down that aisle! We've found that *wanting* to be married is the first step on the way to wedded bliss. And we do not mean some fantasy of marriage, but a sincere willingness to embrace the entire commitment. Marriage takes a great deal of patience, commitment, compromise, sharing, growth, sacrifice, passion, understanding, giving, taking, tolerance, humor, tears, sweat, tenacity, and, not least of all, love. If you don't really want to get married, please don't try and "wing it" just for the hell of it. It won't fly. At least, not *forever!* If you've thought long and hard about taking on this difficult task, and still think you *want* to try your hand at being a wife, then you need to determine your *readiness.* Wanting to be married and being ready must go hand in hand. We'll help you determine your actual readiness in Phase I. But only you can truthfully determine if you wholeheartedly *want* to get married.

Let's address one of the biggest problems that seems to be stopping you gals before you even get started: The notion that since you are such a fierce, powerful force to be reckoned with, there's no one out there for you. There's a popular belief that since you're putting so much energy into successfully slammin' this "man's world," you can't attract a Black man that can handle you. *Bull!* Stop turning all of your assets into stumbling blocks. Get this notion out of your head. There are powerful Black men out there looking for *you*. We are here to tell you that part of this problem is in your head and the other part is in the media's (not so subliminal) messages about our men. You've been brainwashed into believing that there are only a small number of Black men doing great things. Well, maybe according to the TV, but according to our latest survey, there are lots of successful Black men (maybe even a million) out there who are lonely and looking for someone to marry.

In other words, don't be so picky. If you are looking for "Prince Charming," get real. Are you really "Princess Diva"? Remember that marriage takes two people. If you've been gettin' a lot of things your way, this is not how a happy union materializes. Don't get caught in the trap of thinking that you're supposed to find someone to put you on a pedestal. A little modesty goes a long way. We're not saying lower your standards for who is right for you, just be realistic.

You need to realize how much of what you *want* is actually what you *need*. Understanding this distinction is the way to dissolve the myth that you're so powerful that you won't find Mr. Right. He's out there. Trust us, we know how to find him, hook him, and trap him. And while you're at it, trust yourself! Because guess what? *You* know how to find him too. You just don't know it yet! We have created a program that requires *you* to come to terms with vital information about *your* life. You are the only one who knows what you've been doing wrong. It's time to face facts and stop avoiding the inevitable. Own up to your misgivings about your attractiveness and wifely capabilities. Stop doubting yourself. You are a warm, loving person who deserves to find an equally warm, loving person to call your very own. It's not as hard as it seems. We'll help you figure out where your strengths lie as well as figure out what mistakes you might be repeating. A positive attitude about your own successfulness is a tremendous asset in achieving any goal. From now on the glass is *always half full,* OK?

In case you are wondering how we developed this foolproof plan, it was out of a desire to get married and have children. We realized that just because we were career womben, that didn't mean that finding a husband was old-fashioned or unempowering. In fact, we saw that just the opposite was possible. Self-empowerment has never tasted so sweet.

No, we haven't spelled the word *womban/womben* (the *b* is silent) wrong. It's a spelling that we consciously chose to make the word separate unto itself, instead of a deviation from the word *man.* In honor of our Black Foremothers of wombanist philosophy such as Sojourner Truth, Fannie Lou Hamer, Angela Davis, Shirley Chisholm, Coretta Scott King, bell hooks, Dr. Betty Shabazz, Patricia Williams, and Alice Walker, we chose to use an alternate spelling. We hope that you too will feel the amazing exhilaration that accompanies self-actualization when faced with life's everyday challenges (such as looking for a husband).

If you've reached a point in your life where you feel like you've become desperate, don't despair, we've all been there. Don't beat yourself up. Don't focus on the things you have no control over. Instead put all of your energies into the things you can change. The right man will come along when you're ready. A lot of you have stayed in dead-end jobs, in hopes of finding a man who would "change" everything! This is not going to happen. It's never too late to assert yourself. If you take a deep breath and make those hard decisions you've been avoiding, you might just be surprised at how it all turns out. We assure you that if you don't take risks concerning your own happiness, you will never be able to take the risk of marrying "The One."

As the adage teaches us, good luck is preparation meeting opportunity. Your success rests on how prepared you are to be a wife when you finally meet your future husband. You might think that your "herstory" of unsuccessful relationships, past emotional trauma, and other faults is what's keeping you from finding a suitable mate; instead, you should be thinking that all of your herstory can be transformed into a "positive you." Suffice it to say that no matter what you think your social "flaws" may be, there is a Black man out there who will love you and be willing to commit to you in spite of, or maybe even because of, your unique differences. Just use this program to complete the transformation to becoming a *Mrs.*

Remember, as a Black Womban your strength and power lie in your ability to create. Put that energy to use by creating the life that *you* want. Essentially, you must first grant yourself the freedom to imagine yourself as an ideal wife before you can begin the transformation necessary to actually become her. We sanction your right to give yourself permission to figure out exactly who this person is. We affirm that a wombanist philosophy is essential in the process of marrying a Black man and having a happy marriage.

We acted on this realization when I, Cassandra, was several months pregnant with my second child, by my second husband. I hadn't really even wanted to get married again. It just happened! Monique decided that she was ready to get married and asked me how it had happened for me. I told her that even though I hadn't consciously thought about getting married, I had changed the way I had been doing things in my life without really knowing it. I explained that since I wasn't interested in getting married again, I seemed cool and carefree to my husband-to-be. She proceeded to pick my brain to see just how I'd bagged Elmer. The more I thought about it, the more pieces of advice surfaced in my brain. Monique started to get the hang of this process of metamorphosing into a Mrs. As a result of our collaborative efforts and ideas, we devised this foolproof program that transformed Monique into the happily married Mrs. Robert deJongh Jr. in under six months. (Although it may take you longer.) After numerous inquiries from single girlfriends as to how we pulled this off, our "secret" program became the premise for this book.

You will find that our book is a concise, witty, self-help workbook/manual/journal written in our original tongue-in-cheek Africentric vernacular, with African-print borders designed by Monique, original poetry by Cassandra, healing meditations by both of us, and original illustrations by cartoonist Barbara Brandon. Barbara, the first nationally syndicated Black female cartoonist, humorously caricatures us, while highlighting key ideas throughout the book. We hope you are at a point in your life where you are ready to take our advice to heart. We suggest that you give yourself at least two years to make it all happen. If you turn out to be as lucky as Monique was, all the better. But real change doesn't happen overnight. It usually takes time. And only you can tell what changes you need to make to find your husband. Are you willing to do the work needed to get the job done? If you are, then it's a piece of *wedding* cake!

INTRODUCTION

MAKIN' IT ALL WORK FOR YOU

Are you ready to create your own program?   **Y N**

Are you ready to take your life into your own hands?   **Y N**

Are you ready to find your husband?   **Y N**

That's just what we've accomplished. *You can too!*

Are you ready to create your own program?   **Y N**

Are you ready to take your life into your own hands?   **Y N**

Are you ready to find your husband?   **Y N**

That's just what we've accomplished. *You can too!*

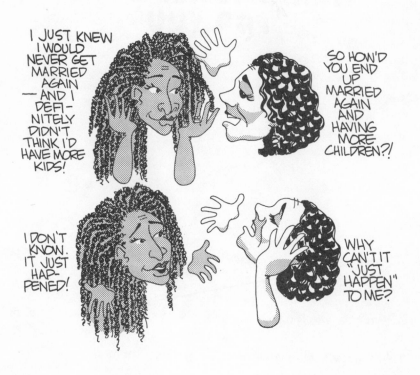

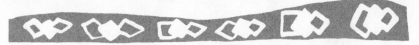

How to Use This Book

Use this book to develop your own personal program for finding a husband. Read and absorb the information here and vigorously apply it to yourself. Answer the soul-searching questions and do the meditations and the exercises that force you to face the only real obstacle between you and marriage: *you!* We firmly believe that if you adapt this program to meet your needs, you will find that the only thing standing between you and your husband is time—the necessary time that it will take you to transform from the single career partygirl diva that you are now into the Mrs. you are destined to become. You've already made the initial investment by buying this book. Continue the commitment to yourself by being honest and tenacious.

How to Marry a Black Man is easy if you realize how wonderful Black men can be. Black men can be warm, funny, strong, dependable, consistent, understanding, intelligent, honest, ambitious, earnest, caring, sexy, romantic, loving, and a *gazillion* other wonderful things. Black men possess an indescribable creative flair that changes everything they come into contact with. Our Black men have worked hard toward solving their most basic survival needs—keeping themselves and their culture alive—while simultaneously and ingeniously satisfying the dominant culture's needs. By relying on humor and wit to get us through the rough spots, Black men manage to focus on what's really important. This ability to bypass petty nonsense and get down to the *real nitty gritty* is essentially the secret of their survival. Black men are still fighting the odds—they have survived amazing trials and rage so overwhelming that we cringe at the idea of the challenges they've overcome. Our praises are not nearly jubilant and supportive enough to celebrate their accomplishments.

Their seemingly endless original interpretations of life continue to tantalize the opposite sex. The richness and depth of the Black man has evoked curiosity throughout the millennia. They have satisfied, and continue to satisfy, our sweet romantic feminine yearnings. As for the Black man's sexual techniques, let's just say that the variations span a soulful range that begins as a whisper, builds to a roar, and ends in a sigh. Intellect, combined with humor and creativity, has always been an unbeatable combination of the Black male survivalist. Black men are greatly sought after and cherished by Black womben.

We think that womben who can be classified as "Wild Womben"—independent, outrageous, career-minded, etc.— should wait until they are in their thirties to marry. That way they have plenty of time and opportunity to explore themselves, life, and the world. More sedate, settled womben who are practically born knowing what they want can marry at an earlier age; but no younger than twenty-five—they still need to plan and save a little something for the future.

How to Marry a Black Man is a manual that is divided into three phases. Use it like a journal—it's cheaper than therapy. Throughout, we've asked questions and supplied spaces for you to write in answers; there are also some blank pages at the end of the book. It's a permanent record of your thoughts and feelings which will reflect your personal growth. It's portable and will always be available even when you have no one to talk to.

If you use it consistently, you will begin to recognize your patterns of growth and maturity. It becomes quite reassuring to see your own development progress toward a positive goal. Give yourself adequate time to accomplish your goals.

The first phase boosts self-awareness, the second phase motivates physical action, and the third phase inspires reflection. Please complete each phase before you move on to the next one. You can read this book in one sitting, but you cannot complete the program in one reading. It will change your mindset and put you well on the road to matrimony. As you will see, our workbook will *motivate* you.

Once you've bagged your Brothah, share your book with him. Get his thoughts and feelings about the issues we raise. Make sure he answers some of the questions, not only the ones designed for him, but also any that you think might lead to an interesting or important conversation.

At the beginning of each chapter, check out the "Word from the Brothahs" boxes. We arranged dozens of all-male focus groups and interviews in which black men spoke out for themselves about what they really want from Black womben. The boxes contain surprising quotations from the down-to-earth Brothahs (aged twenty-five to seventy) whom we've interviewed—the kind of Brothahs that *you* want to marry. We reveal what Black men *really* think and feel about relationships that lead to marriage with Sistahs. Heed what they have to say.

If you're serious about wanting to marry a Black man, take our quiz, "Twenty-Five Questions . . . and Then Some," and if you're *ready, willing,* and *able*—start *your* program.

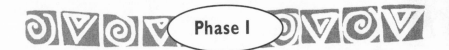

GETTIN' YOURSELF
TOGETHAH

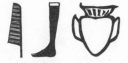

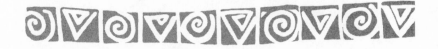

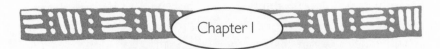
TWENTY-FIVE QUESTIONS . . . AND THEN SOME

Word from the Brothahs

If I could give all single Black womben a message, what would it be?

"Take your time. Take your time! Don't rush into anything. There are a lot of good Black brothers out there. And there are a million of us who are trying to do the right thing. But don't oversimplify, don't prejudge us because we are Black. "Develop yourself."

"If the brother is not showing you respect, kindness, consideration, interest, and all that kind of stuff right up front, this is a brother that you need to stay away from."

Many of you might be thinking, "I'm not married because I can't meet Mr. Right." But we believe you probably have met him. It's just that deep down inside, you believe that you don't deserve him. *We know you do!*

This is a how-to book in its most basic form. We give you questions to get you thinking about various areas of your life that contribute to your relationships, and we offer concise, constructive instructions. If you're a shy, quiet, withdrawn person, you must decide if you're willing to change your modus operandi to find and marry a Black man. Unless you throw your entire being into makin' it happen, our program may not work for you.

Are You Ready? . . .

Before you continue reading, set aside some quiet time and take our twenty-five-question self-assessment quiz. This quiz gauges five aspects of your personality: spirituality, emotional stability, mental health, physical health, and cultural awareness. If you've been married before, please take this quiz as well as answering the questions in Chapter X (pp. 191–212). Please reflect honestly before answering, and be decisive: "maybe" or "sometimes" is scored as a "No" answer.

Are You Ready Spiritually?

1. Are you centered? Do you feel whole and complete in your soul? **Y N**
2. Do you have a good, solid relationship with your Creator/the Universe? **Y N**
3. Do you recognize positive energy that comes to you from close friends and relatives? **Y N**
4. Do you nourish your soul with natural beauty and positive people? **Y N**
5. Are you aware of the power of focused positive energy in your world? **Y N**

Are You Ready Mentally?

6. Are you aware of how your decision-making process works? **Y N**
7. Do you express yourself clearly to others? **Y N**
8. Can you be bold, flexible, and decisive? **Y N**
9. Do you have any hobbies or interests outside your job? **Y N**
10. Are you willing to take advice in order to meet, greet, and keep a man? **Y N**

Are You Ready Emotionally?

11. Have you ever been in love? **Y N**
12. Do you love yourself completely? **Y N**

13. Do you have ongoing loving, committed relationships with others? **Y N**

14. Can you tell the difference between true love and infatuation? **Y N**

15. Can you love unconditionally? **Y N**

Are You Ready Physically?

16. Have you had varied sexual experiences? **Y N**

17. Are you clear about your sexual orientation? **Y N**

18. Are you happy with your body the way it is? **Y N**

19. Are you where you want to be in life? **Y N**

20. Have you had an AIDS test? **Y N**

Are You Ready Culturally?

21. Do you know that our culture's herstory/history is not accurately represented in most educational systems? **Y N**

22. Are you aware of the varied social, scientific, and literary contributions made to our society by African Americans? **Y N**

23. Are you aware of the hopelessness voiced in some of our young people's music? **Y N**

24. Do you actively seek ways to empower yourself and your family and friends? **Y N**

25. A new Black Renaissance has emerged in our community. Have you read any Black scholarly work in the last year? **Y N**

Scoring and Working It All Out

If you answered "No" to:
A. 0 questions: You are ready.
B. 1 to 5: You're almost ready.
C. 6 to 12: You're *not* ready.
D. 13 or more: Don't even think about getting married ... yet!

Remember: "Maybe" or "Sometimes" are scored as "No" answers.

A. If you have answered "Yes" to most or all of the twenty-five questions, then you are ready to follow our program and are seriously ready to get married. We only ask that you follow our program explicitly and give it your all.

B. If you answered "No" to five or fewer questions, you still have some work to do on making yourself a complete, happy, and mature womban ready for commitment.

C. If you answered "No" to six to twelve questions, you have a lot of other questions to answer, beginning with "Why do you want to get married in the first place?" A careful and deep soul search will probably bring up issues that you have not dared look at before. Take it easy on yourself. Go slowly. There really is no rush. The only constraints you have are the ones you place on yourself.

D. If you answered "No" to thirteen or more questions, you're not close to knowing yourself, never mind knowing who you want to marry. You need to look closely and carefully at your motivations for seeking matrimony. Remember, marrying someone to make up for something lacking in yourself is not a good move. It actually stunts your growth.

Note: If most of your "No" answers are in one category, you are probably neglecting one aspect of your personality. This doesn't mean that you're a hopeless case; it simply means that you have some work to do to get yourself ready for that march down the aisle.

Many people are not able to answer "Yes" to all of these questions by their Wedding Day, but through the caring, sharing, and growing that marriage entails, they will continue to develop the best of themselves. And that's what this book is about—getting yourself ready to "jump the broom." ('Cause let's face it, if you knew what to do and how to do it, you wouldn't need this book!)

Now that you've scored your quiz, the next few pages will help you focus on specific areas where you might be out of balance. In addition to answering the questions we pose here, it's a good idea to keep journal entries recording your progress at integrating this information into your life. This process of growth requires that you spend time thinking, expanding your reading, and getting out into the world. You need to change the way you think about Black men and marriage.

Your Spiritual Life

Get in tune, Sis. If you answered "No" to one or more of these questions, then you need to get centered. You are trying to find someone to complement you, not complete you. A committed, serious relationship with your creator, Goddess, spiritual forces (or whatever you choose to call that Universal Energy) will give you the freedom to live and enjoy your life exactly as it is.

One way to provide nourishment for your soul is to become

more aware of the natural beauty in your surroundings. Another way is to surround yourself with positive people—they will uplift your spirits just by being around them. Try and steer clear of negative people who criticize and complain about everything (even if they are close to you). Begin to think positively and be a positive person—you need to develop and recognize positivity in yourself before you can recognize it in a potential husband. Positivity attracts positivity. Nothing is as attractive as a happy, complete womban.

Which aspects of your spiritual life satisfy you most and why?

_____

_____

_____

_____

What if anything is lacking in your spiritual life?

_____

_____

_____

_____

How can you increase your spiritual awareness on a daily basis?

_____

_____

_____

_____

Your Mental Processes

You need to know how to make decisions and be aware of how you make them before you can decide what you want in a man. And you need intellectual stimulation—in the form of hobbies, classes, or political or social involvement—to help keep you alert and interesting. You will also meet guys by getting out and getting involved. In order to follow our program, Sistah, you must be bold!

What is it about making decisions that causes you anxiety?

_____

_____

_____

_____

What is the worst thing that could happen if you make the wrong decision? _____

_____

_____

_____

Can you accept responsibility for the consequences of your decisions?

_____

If yes, how? _____

_____

_____

_____

If not, why?

_____

_____

_____

_____

List some of your interests outside of your job.

_____

_____

_____

_____

What good advice have you incorporated into your life lately?

_____

_____

_____

_____

What can you do to change your style of communication so that peo-ple understand you better?

_____

_____

_____

_____

Do you feel that many of your conversations with Black men end in misunderstandings? If so, why?

_____

_____

_____

_____

Your Emotional Stability

You have to love yourself unconditionally if you expect someone else to love you in the same way. Committed, loving relationships with family and friends are a training ground for your life-long commitment to a spouse. Mending or releasing yourself from negative relationships with family and friends can open your heart to more loving connections.

If you've never been in love or experienced true love, then you may have some emotional blocks that can be alleviated by group counseling, therapy, or womben's support groups. You may have experienced infatuation—a self-indulgent, one-sided, intense emotion that can easily be mistaken for true love. It is usually physical and sexual in nature. The real person's needs, wants, and personality are obscured by your desire to fit him into your fantasy mold. True love is mutual, based on knowing and understanding each other's good *and* bad qualities.

List a few things that you love about yourself.

_____

_____

Name some people that you love and why. (Pets can be included in this list.)

_____

_____

Define unconditional love.

_____

_____

Describe a situation when you feel you were infatuated with someone.

_____

_____

_____

_____

_____

If you have experienced love, how did it differ from infatuation?

_____

_____

_____

_____

_____

Where is love lacking in your life?

_____

_____

Your Physical Well-being

It's your body, baby. If you don't worship your body as a temple, how do you expect someone else to. It doesn't matter what your body looks like, as long as you've developed and consistently follow an exercise program. As long as you're healthy and in good shape, learn to love and accept yourself as you are. If you can't, then consider individual or group therapy to help you develop a positive self-image. Remember, even three can form a group. Don't be discouraged; not being where you want to be in life can be a great motivator. It can provide you with ambition, focus, and a burning interest in achieving a certain goal. These qualities can be very attractive to an ambitious, focused Black man.

Some of you may have experimented sexually, some may not have. Questioning your sexuality is normal and healthy. If you still have questions or issues, now is the time to deal with them. Just make sure that you've had whatever sexual experiences you wanted before "settlin' down."

What do you like best about your body? _____

Least? _____

Which sexual experiences would you like to repeat?

_____

_____

Why or why not?

_____

_____

_____

_____

_____

Which sexual experiences would you never even think of again?

_____

_____

What sexual experience (if any) would you like to have that you haven't already tried?

_____

_____

What steps do you have to take to be where you want to be in your life both physically and sexually?

_____

_____

_____

_____

_____

_____

The AIDS Test

In this day and age, any sexually active person who is looking for a mate should have an AIDS test. This way if you turn up positive, you are not starting a relationship in confusion. We encourage you to seek information, counseling, and support groups about living with HIV. You can deal with the ramifications of the situation before you get into a relationship. If results are negative, you'll have the peace of mind necessary to pursue your goal. In either case you'll have a vested interest in practicing safer sex.

Caution: *Do not let a negative test result be an excuse for not practicing Safer Sex. Each and every time you have sex you must use a condom.*

If you have not been tested, what are your fears? List them. If you have been tested, when and why do you plan to retest?

Your Cultural Life

The truth shall set you free. Having a strong identification with your cultural roots can only empower you. Much of our his/herstory has been masterfully manipulated to reflect half-truths that intentionally and purposefully emasculate our Brothahs. As you uncover the truths, through research and self-reeducation, you will experience a cultural metamorphosis that feeds your soul, your mind, and your raison d'être. Black men want to attach themselves to womben who are on the move and know what time it is.

There is great joy in taking pride in yourself and where you live, no matter how meager your life and surroundings may seem. Remember, it's not where you live, but how you live! Hope will be restored to us all with the understanding that having money is not all it's cracked up to be. We must focus on the importance of possessing integrity, pride, and intelligence. It's not entirely your fault for focusing on financial success. Don't be too hard on yourself. You were a Buppie seed your parents planted in hopes of raising a well-equipped and financially successful person.

Hope results from the knowledge that there were other periods of his/herstory when not only did we control the game, but there existed Black civilizations so fierce that most of the "inventions" of modern civilization were stolen and/or adapted from these "conquered," ancient societies. Factually, a well-kept secret. Black people with this knowledge have the power!

For further enlightenment on the his/herstory of our culture, you can turn to works by formidable scholars and visionaries such as Ivan Van Sertima, Dr. John H. Clark, Dr. Ben Joachannan,

Cornel West, Nikki Giovanni, Maya Angelou, Ntozake Shange, bell hooks, and Molefi Kete Asante . . . to name just a few. (See Bibliography.)

Can you name additional visionaries or scholars?

_____

_____

List some of your more inspiring influences to date.

_____

_____

List three cultural events you intend to participate in within the next few months.

_____

_____

One of the most affirming ways to recapture the true impact of ancient African contributions to our Western civilization is to actually visit Egypt or any other of the African nations. Have you (or has anyone in your family) been to the Motherland?　　**Y　N**

If you have been so fortunate, describe your jubilation at seeing our people in their native land.

_____

_____

_____

_____

If you have the chance, visit any (so-called) Third World country once dominated by any European power and witness for yourself the legacy left by that desiccating power. Seek to find the differences between the "native" way of life and the tourist attractions. Have you been to any of these places? If so, describe your reactions to experiencing the results of European domination.

_____

_____

_____

_____

You've done good work so far. This is just the beginning of the process of becoming ready for marriage. Now that you're doing everything in your power to better yourself, the next step is to accept your own imperfections. No one is perfect. Having a healthy respect for your own human frailties is an important key to allowing yourself to "Say 'I Do' to You."

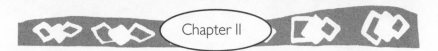

Chapter II

SAY "I DO" TO YOU!

Word from the Brothahs

"You can't expect somebody to love you if you don't love yourself."

"When you're with somebody, you have to be able to... look at that person, strip them naked, and boil them down to their essence. And say to yourself, can you embrace that essence?... If you can't embrace that essence, you shouldn't be with that person."

What makes a womban marriage material?

"My checklist in a womban I'd like to marry? I want a womban with an education... with lots and lots of self-esteem. The desire to move upwards. The desire to become better than you were when I met you. You know, I want growth. I want honesty, sincerity. Because this is what I'm willing to give. And I will only give it because I believe it's what I'm going to get back."

"I'm not terribly religious myself but I want a womban who has values... to be sincere and honest... a pretty well rounded person...to also have a wild side...and [be] spiritual....Like I said, I'm not a very religious person, but I consider myself [to be] a spiritual person. I believe there are certain things that you can create inside yourself spiritually, energy-wise, to help yourself."

"For me? The bottom line is...what I'm willing to give, I want back...honesty, integrity, strength. Intelligence."

"The person who may be right for you or who may have an interest in you may pass by while you're beating yourself over the head about somebody who doesn't [give a damn about you]."

"There's a lot of desperate sisters out there who will take abuse and the Brothers know that."

"You want a womban who can think on her feet. Fearless."

"Right. You want a womban that can function...if something happened...a crisis happened...she can handle it...and can handle it in a way in which you would want it handled."

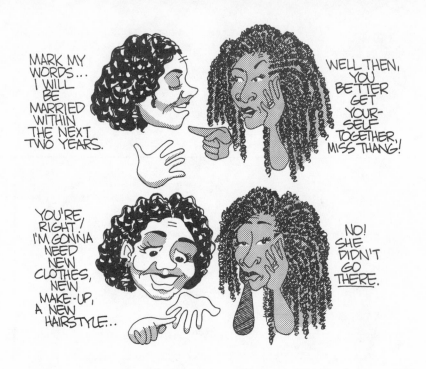

Before entering into marriage, we wholeheartedly believe that before you say "I do" to someone else, you must first make a commitment to yourself. You have to believe with your mind, body, and soul that you *want* to get married. You must believe that you are worthy and ready for marriage. This sounds simple, but it isn't. You have to make certain vows to *yourself* before you can make these promises to him.

Nuptials for One

These things I promise myself:

I will be faithful to and honest with myself;

I will respect, trust, help, and care for myself;

I will live my life for me, fully;

I will forgive myself;

I will try to better understand myself, the world, and God—

through the best and worst of what is to come, as long as I live.

Do you solemnly swear to heal your heart so that it can be open to new love? _____ I do.

Do you solemnly swear to forgive yourself for the mistakes you've made? _____ I do.

Do you solemnly swear to remain chaste for an extended time? _____ I do.

Do you solemnly swear to fully release former emotional attachments? _____ I do.

Do you solemnly swear to say affirmations every day? _____ I do.

Do you solemnly swear, as a widow, to release the guilt that restricts you? _____ I do.

Do you solemnly swear to create a five-year plan and stick to it? _____ I do.

Do you solemnly swear to allow yourself to love and be loved again? _____ I do.

Vow of Self-healing

This is an exercise devised by Shakti Gawain and related by Donna Cunningham in her book *Healing Pluto Problems*. You can adapt this exercise for use on any of the seven chakras, spiraling centers of energy located throughout the body; it is given here for the heart chakra. Spiritualists use these vital energy centers as a map to explore who we are, how we got the way we are, and what we can do to become who we want to be. The heart chakra is of primary importance in opening us up to more loving relationships and mending old hurts and losses. Many people have suffered damage to the heart center. The exercise uses an affirmation, the repetition of a key phrase that relates to the center in question. An affirmation can also be used to open other chakras; it is important to open and cleanse all the centers equally to avoid creating an imbalance.

The Heart Flower Meditation

To begin, mentally place yourself in a bubble. Imagine your heart center as a beautiful many-petaled flower, with the petals closed. A positive color for the flower would be bright pink, since that is the color of love. Starting at the outside, open the petals, one by one. With each petal, affirm your willingness to give and receive love. You may do it by saying inwardly, "I am open to love," or whatever seems pleasing to you. Actually moving your hands through your energy field as if you were opening the petals greatly increases the effect. Keep opening petals and opening petals and opening petals, while steadily repeating the affirmation. As you near the center, notice that the petals are glowing with pink light, which is warm to the touch. When the center itself is open, the pink light radiates from it and pulsates outward past the edge of your bubble. Say to yourself, "This light from my heart is a beacon to those who would rightfully share love with me." Draw down pink light from your Higher Self to send outward.

This exercise is a powerful one. You may find it somewhat difficult at first, as the pain you are carrying in your heart center may surface. Yet allowing it to come up, thawing out, and releasing the grief it entails is an important part of the process of healing yourself. As you repeat this exercise, you will notice movement and energy in your heart. When someone you care about comes around, you will notice an outward rush of energy from the heart that feels uplifting. The heart chakra is quite sensitive and may close down easily when someone around you is insensitive or does something to hurt you. It may also close down in self-protection. When it's closed, you will notice the absence of those heart rushes and know that it is time to work the exercise again.

Following is a blank page for you to record observations of your reactions to the exercise. Write down any of the positive or negative feelings that came up while you were doing the exercise; and then decide how you want to deal with them.

Heart Flower Exercise

_____

_____

_____

_____

_____

_____

_____

_____

_____

_____

_____

_____

_____

_____

Vow of Forgiveness

If you forgive yourself for past mistakes that have caused you pain in loving, you can allow greater happiness to enter and transform your life forever.

I am sorry my old lover(s) hurt me.

I forgive myself for allowing it to happen.

I will use my pain as a sword to sever my connection with him.

A good way to start healing old wounds from previous relationships is to free yourself from any emotional/spiritual connections that you are still holding on to. By first forgiving yourself for having been involved, you allow yourself the opportunity to genuinely attract a new partner. If you don't forgive yourself, this may never happen.

For some of you, therapy or group support might be necessary to help you accomplish self-forgiveness. There are plenty of Sistahs out there who are in the same boat as you. If you can't afford therapy, or just aren't into it, you should get together with a couple of positive, powerful Sistahs and start getting your heads together. Talk to one another about your hang-ups. Do some real soul searching about how you keep sabotaging yourselves. Encourage emotional support for one another. Bolster your friends' vulnerable areas. Don't turn these gatherings into *bitch* sessions, where all you do is complain about the state of your lives. Use the time constructively to examine your own weak points and learn to accept feedback. Listen carefully to what the other Sistahs are saying to you. Try to learn from their mistakes and your own. If you work hard, you'll see positive results.

Vow of Celibacy

Abstain from sex for a while and concentrate on yourself. By abstaining from intercourse, you will gather all of your sexual energy inside yourself. A dynamic sexual force will fill you completely and exude through every pore. Consider this energy your life force. Feel its substance. The amount of sexual energy that you develop will be a magnet to single men. The right man will find your sexual energy irresistible. If you have truly detached yourself from *all* old lovers, this energy will provide a channel for "The One" to locate you.

End all "fuck-buddy" relationships—you know what we mean! Discontinue any relationships that are purely sexual. Having casual lovers is fine if that's what you want. But if you're looking for a permanent relationship—a husband—these casual affairs only distract you from finding the right man.

Vow to Release Obsessive Fixations

If you are currently in or trying to get over an obsessive relationship, you must take heart in knowing that you *can* and *must* get him out of your system. It's imperative that you release yourself from the energy that has you captive. Cut the ties that bind you to him.

Note: If this relationship is either physically or emotionally abusive, seek professional help immediately!

Make a list of all the terrible and not so terrible things he did to you over the course of your relationship.

_____

_____

_____

_____

Write down the last time he made you cry and why.

_____

_____

_____

Add to the list every time he's made you angry.

_____

_____

_____

Look at the list you've just created. What part did you play in letting your emotions get the best of your better judgment?

_____

_____

_____

_____

Why aren't you able to let him go?

_____

_____

_____

_____

What is it gonna take to convince you that he is not "The One"?

_____

_____

_____

_____

Is the scenario you outlined above one that you would like to see fulfilled? **Y N**

How will you release yourself from this attachment?

_____

_____

_____

_____

Let go of the idea that he is the only man on earth who can fulfill your needs. Heaven forbid you should still have a physical relationship with him on any level, but if you do, *for goodness' sake, stop sleeping with the guy!* Cutting out sex won't guarantee that your obsession will end. But it will force you to see the other parts of his personality and to face the reality that you're in a dead-end relationship.

He doesn't want you in the way that you want to be wanted. He does, however, want to know that you are under his magic spell; that is, his ego wants all your attention and your loving care, for little or nothing in return. He *may* seem to be reciprocating your level of interest, but if this were true, he would be into you as much as you're into him . . . *all of the time,* not just when he feels the urge. The quality of attention and romance he bestows on you is intense when he does show interest, right? But it's inconsistent at best. Stop pouring all of your energy into a bottomless pit. The good qualities that this guy may have are available in other men. Start looking for positive qualities in a different man. This is a challenge to your personal growth, but we know you can and will find a more suitable man.

Vow of Daily Affirmations

Create an affirmation for yourself, such as

> *I deserve to be treated well at all times.*

or

> *I am worthy of allowing a wonderful Black man into my life.*

or

> *I only need one single Black man who'll marry me.*

Write down your affirmation(s):

_____

_____

_____

_____

_____

Don't forget to say your affirmation(s) *every day* or as often as you can remember to. Write down your affirmations and then put them in prominent places throughout your home. An affirmation taped to your bedroom or bathroom mirror or your refrigerator serves as a handy reminder. The affirmations will allow you to consider and appreciate the possibilities for growth in your life. You should write new ones or revise the affirmations as your life starts to change.

Another affirmation you might want to try is

The right Black man will come into my life at the right time.

Vow to Release Guilt

Meditation for Widows

I see my deceased loved one in the glow of a heavenly light,

Peacefully enjoying his favorite activities.

I imagine him watching over me shining the light of his love

before me, on my path.

I take solace in knowing that he wants me to be happy again.

I release myself from the guilt I feel for wanting a new love.

I deserve happiness and what I ask for, he will help me

to receive.

If you are a widow or have lost your mate, you *can* find love again. Learn to respect your own needs and desires; they are normal and healthy. You can still keep a small piece of him in your heart forever—just allow a new part to be discovered. Force yourself to do the things that encourage you to reach out for spiritual nourishment. Read, meditate, dance, listen to the wind. It tells a secret only you can hear: that you are free of pain; that your memories together will help you find a new love to travel through life with. Feel your grief without wallowing in it. Don't forget that you are still alive. Don't waste precious time and energy. We can't tell you *exactly* what to do, because everyone mourns differently, but allow your own heart to guide you. Just when you think you can't take anymore, the grief usually starts to let up. Ask for divine guidance and seek support from family and friends. You *will* find peace.

Vow to Create a Five-Year Plan

We suggest that you sit down and actually write a letter of intent to yourself: *a five-year plan.* Describe in detail what you want for yourself and how you intend to get it. Include career goals as well as personal goals. After much reflection, develop a strategy. Then make a vow to follow the plan; solemnly swear to see it through. Writing it down makes a difference, imprinting it into your subconscious. Then, in five years, you can compare what you actually accomplished with what you vowed to do. If you say "I do" to you, you'll be surprised at how many dreams come true.

My Five-Year Plan

In the next five years, I do solemnly swear to

_____

_____

_____

_____

_____

_____

_____

_____

_____

_____

_____

_____

These vows to yourself are more important than anything you might pledge to someone else. You must establish a pattern of looking inside yourself to determine what your next course of action will be to achieve your goals, in the long and the short term. If you haven't the slightest idea what you need, how are you going to determine what you have to do to get it? This kind of personal goal setting must become a part of your daily mental housekeeping. You should determine what your goals are. It's been proven that people who set low standards and unchallenging goals have a lower success rate at reaching any goals. However, people who set high standards for themselves usually reach their goals. So reach for the stars. Then backtrack and figure out what steps you need to take to move in that direction.

By embarking on an ongoing, enlightening spiritual journey, you can familiarize yourself with methods of tapping into the positively magical sources of self-renewal. Prayer, yoga, meditation, affirmations, singing, dancing, Tai Chi, swimming, and nature walks are all methods of self-renewal. All of these activities will allow you to bring your contemplative focused skills into play. Daily affirmations, words, and rituals reinforce the light within and enhance your physical, spiritual, and emotional beauty.

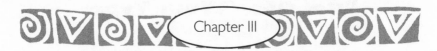
NOT YOUR "TYPE"

Word from the Brothahs

"She said to me that her biological time clock is ticking, and 'I want a corny guy now.'"

Corny guy? What's a corny guy?

"How do you define corny? What is corny? Well, I guess corny to womben is a guy who can say to his girl...honestly, 'Look, I don't want nobody else, baby, all I want is you.' Okay, that's corny...nowadays."

"I think the message would be to approach each situation as new...you know, as an individual, brand-new situation. If there's one thing I hate, it's to be judged by a womban's past with other men. I hate that. Because that just doesn't do me any justice at all."

So what if he's not your type! How well have you been treated by the "type" of guy you've been dating? You have to release the image of the "Perfect Man" and do a reality check. Looks can be deceiving.

"Get Over" Your Type

"Go out with almost any guy who doesn't make you sick."

This was Cassandra's advice to Monique, and it worked for both of us. We're not suggesting that you compromise on your criteria for an appropriate mate. It's just that for the purposes of broadening your sensibilities about the "type" of Black man your husband may actually end up being, you should make some (slightly extreme) adjustments about who you turn down for dates . . . at least for the next few months. You have to shock yourself out of your lifelong idea that only a certain type of man is appropriate for you. This is an essential step in the process of opening yourself up to meeting Black men who may end up marrying you. You'd be surprised at how many guys are looking for someone just to talk to and hang out with. Leaving yourself open to such an encounter just might lead to something serious.

What is your "type" anyway?

_____

_____

_____

_____

If you don't know what your "type" is or if you're having a problem figuring out what it is, try this: Imagine you've arrived at a party (fashionably late, of course), looking hot, and you start scoping the room to see what's happenin'. Describe the "type" of guy that catches your eye and sends chills up your spine:

_____

_____

_____

_____

This is who you should *stay away from,* at least for a while. While that music is making you wish *anyone* would ask you to dance, give the other Brothahs a chance to ask you. Smile and flirt with someone who isn't your "type." See what happens.

That's what I, Monique, did. I met my husband at a disco. Unbelievable, right? No one ever meets anyone decent at a nightclub, right? Not! (He was, however, introduced to me by a mutual friend.) The first thing I noticed about him was that he wasn't my "type." The next thing I noticed was that he was better than my "type"—cause he was flirting with *me* (and he *was* cute in his own way). If I had stuck to my "type," I would have missed out on the most romantic Black man I've ever known. So see, girls, you gotta let go of that "type" and get ready to meet your husband-to-be!

What is the opposite of your "type"?

_____

_____

_____

_____

_____

These are the kinds of guys you should have an open mind about. It may take you a little while to let go of your firmly fastened beliefs. But that's OK! This transformation is not going to happen overnight. Trust yourself to know when and how fast to assimilate all of this new information about other types of guys into your life.

There is a difference between your *needs* and your *wants*. Your *needs* evolve from listening to your inner voice assessing your values and understanding your life experiences. These needs may include the desire for home, family, partnership, companionship, and love.

Your *wants* are usually a reaction to outside influences, e.g., family, friends, the media, and public opinion. Your wants may involve unrealistic notions about romance, excitement, social status, or material benefits. There is a great deal to be said for being able to mesh both needs and wants into one relationship, but try not to confuse the two. You may have been brought up to want a high-powered man when a less driven, more accessible guy is really what you need. You have to learn how to prioritize these similar desires so that your needs are met before your wants are fulfilled.

What do you *want* from a Black man in a relationship?

_____

_____

_____

_____

_____

What do you *need* from a Black man in a relationship?

_____

_____

_____

_____

_____

What are some of your fears?

_____

_____

_____

_____

The key is to determine what your real *needs* are and how to best fulfill them. Sometimes that has to be determined by trial and error. Too many of us go after what we think we want instead of what we need. Our wants and desires have been determined by all of these years of exposure to the media. Don't trust your wants! You should instead trust your gut instincts as to what you *need* to truly be happy in a lifelong committed relationship.

The intangible qualities of understanding, unconditional love, intimate sharing, and intellectual compatibility are *more important* than superficial qualities like looks, image, etc. You must stop limiting your sensibilities unnecessarily. Just because he looks sexy, handsome, and cool doesn't mean he is loving, patient, and committed, as a husband must be. Looks can be deceiving. Another thing we had to realize was this: Age is a matter of mind—if you don't mind, then it doesn't matter! Opening your mind to a vast range of possibilities is just one of the keys to finding your husband.

It was for me, Monique. Cassandra told me, "Go out with almost any guy that doesn't make you sick!" I thought she was crazy because I always knew that my husband was going to be tall, honey colored (like me), have light-colored eyes, and be a Casanova. So why would I go out with anyone who doesn't look like my "type"? After all, every last one of the guys that fit my personal husband description always broke my heart or sent me into a tizzy. But none of them ever came close to being husband material. None of them wanted to be my husband. They were too busy perfecting their "type."

I was convinced that when I finally found my husband he'd be my "type." Well, he isn't. He's everything else but my "type"— and oh so much more. He's not tall, but he's not short. He's one of the normal, shy, handsome types. He has chocolate-colored skin, deep brown eyes, and he's sweet, kind, and very reliable. He has a nice muscular build without looking like a weightlifter, and, best of all, he loves (almost) everything about me.

Ladies, please don't reject *"normal"* guys as an acceptable type. Normal is good. Normal is great. Normal is what you want to come home to every night. Normal is someone who is there because he's happy and wants to be there.

As a sophisticated career womban *scoping* a *par-tay* for someone to zero in on and flirt with, lots of times you usually pass right over "normal." For some reason there is a strange idea in your head that unless he looks mysterious, cool, or exciting he will be an undesirable mate. Maybe this is true if you're looking for a temporary lover. But if what you want is a husband: Make *normal* your new type!

We both were not really interested in our "normal" guys (our future husbands) when we met them. We were just hangin' out with whoever amused us the most. Then we became charmed by our "normal" guys' manner, intellect, whatever (they both have a lot of excellent qualities!), and let ourselves be pursued. At first glance they didn't appear to be our "types." But as time went by, they both proved with their actions where their hearts were. Genuine interest and caring were their trademarks right from the start. Their *normal* behavior is something we've grown to depend on.

A lack of interest on your part can be a turn-on to a man. *Any man,* no matter what he says. This is one reason it's important to have outside interests and activities—they can keep you from being too "available." But at the same time, don't be so *busy* that you can't squeeze him in "for a few hours," "in a couple of days," or "real soon." If *every* time he thinks of seeing you he has to make an appointment, he'll soon be discouraged.

Note: Allow space for spontaneity. Invite him along. He may prove to be a more willing companion than you anticipated. If he shows interest in you, your life, your thoughts, then why isn't he your "type"?

Be open to all kinds of Black men, especially foreigners. The world is getting smaller every day. You might meet your mate while traveling, taking a course where there are foreign students, on the Internet, living in a college town or a large cosmopolitan area. Just be open to anyone—you never know what will happen!

Also, remember our rule:

Go out with every guy at least two times!

Sometimes a man will seem entirely different on the second date. On the first date he (or you) may have been nervous. Anyone can have a bad day!

He Ain't "All That," Girlfriend!

There are loads of relationship books that will try to steer you away from certain types of men. They will convince you to seek only a select few types of appropriate fellas. We won't.

Instead, we want you to realize one important fact:

All men are capable of behaving like all of the different "types" of Brothahs out there! They can all treat you like "all that and . . ." or "They be doggin' you, baby!"

Many factors—the situation, the developmental stage of both of your lives, your and his readiness for marriage—will influence whether or not you will be "dogged" or treated like a potential wife and mother. We encourage you to look at how he is treating you, because a "dog" can treat you right and a "gentleman" can "dog" you. It all depends . . .

Listen up closely, ladies. You must be able to spot behavior patterns early on, so that you can determine if you're wasting your time or not. Sometimes guys start out with great intentions about how they will behave around you but after taking some cues from how you treat yourself, they change. It all comes back to you. You have more control over this entire process of finding a husband than you know. Soon you will be more aware of just how much power and control you have over your own life.

A man who treats you shamefully can quite easily turn right around and behave extremely courteously to another womban. Conversely, a man that has been touted as a perfect angel can and will act unabashedly roguish around you if you encourage such behavior. Let's make it perfectly clear, however, that your cues are not the only factor that determines his behavior toward you. There are several other reasons that might be influencing his behavior that make him not your type!

Watch for Signs of Unacceptable Behavior

There are certain types of actions when exhibited by men that *ensure* that they are not marriage material. Here are the three major types of unacceptable behavior that you should *stay away from*.

He's not your "type" if he acts like one of the Dogs, Fugitives, or Boyz. Get away from him as quickly as possible, or you're letting yourself in for some heartbreak.

He's Not Your Type. . . . If He Acts like a Dog

Girls, you ought to know better! Once you realize all men can act like dogs, you can usually see them coming from a mile away. If all you want is a good time, by all means engage in a sexy interlude with one of these guys. Just don't go into it blindfolded . . . unless of course it's part of the foreplay. Otherwise, steer clear, if you know what's good for you. Dogs have the ability to manipulate womben into doing things they never thought possible.

This isn't necessarily a bad thing, but beware girls, it *is* "addick-tive"! He may take you on a romantic ride that's (arguably) an escapade that every womban should experience at least once in her life. Then again, we're here to tell you that it ain't that easy to get off the ride.

Beware of the most handsome, seductive, debonair, sweet-talking, smooth-dancing animal you've ever encountered. This kind of Black man possesses a magnetic aura that draws womben to him, like steel filings to a magnet. You can pick him out in a crowd, because he always has womben circling him, waiting to pounce. Since so many womben are throwing themselves at them all the time, Dogs develop a blasé attitude about the hunt, which makes them that much more attractive. What you should realize is that these men suffer the same amount of rejection as the rest of us. They just make it seem like a lot less because so many womben are interested in them in the first place.

Don't let them fool you. A Dog will try to win you over by sharing with you his previous heartbreak(s). As he tells his tall tales, he'll weep great big crocodile tears all over your sensitive, maternal heart, hoping you'll be so distracted that you won't see the sledge hammer poised above your head. He'll lull you into a false sense of security by making you believe that he would *never* do to you what has been done to him. Guess what!?! That's exactly what he'll do. He's mastered the art of nonchalantly inflicting heartache on unsuspecting womben.

Dogs need the illusion of free territory in which to roam. A Dog will run from yard to yard in search of bigger and better bones. You don't want to be a buried bone, never to be thought of again until the lean times come around. Then, he'll be back, sniffing at your back door, scratching and pawing, begging to be let in. Needless to say, if you're serious about getting married, leave the Dogs in the pound! Don't let those big, sad puppy dog eyes coax you into giving him another chance.

He's Not Your Type . . . If He Acts like a Fugitive

The fugitive is always running away from commitment—for various reasons. He may have a serious problem with intimacy, which is slightly different from commitment phobia. In this case, he may indeed decide to marry you, but his emotional makeup may be such that he cannot meet the level of intimate sharing that marriage requires and that you need. Some men have problems sharing their feelings with anyone because they never learned how to get in touch with them in the first place. They face an ongoing challenge to learn how to open up about their life experiences and how to share their emotional reactions to them. This is a lifelong process and many men may never reach the level of sharing that most womben need to maintain lifelong partnerships. If you feel that you've clearly and adequately expressed your dissatisfaction at his inability to be intimate with you, don't hesitate to *move on to the next guy!*

Or maybe he wants to string you along or keep you on the back burner for marriage in the future. Your man is probably trying to achieve a certain level of stability and security, which is one of the hardest things for him to do in our society. Give him a certain amount of time to make a commitment to "settle down," and if he can't or won't, calmly and sweetly inform him that you will be dating other men until he's ready to tie the knot.

The next problem you may face is helping him get over commitment phobia. There are several reasons why Black men fall prey to commitment phobia. It's usually due to a combination of familial upbringing and societal pressures. Men who won't commit have to be handled with care. If you think he's worth it, you may have to prepare yourself to go through the long haul with him. He might not be worth the wait, especially with no guarantee that he'll ever come around. At this point you should tell him, in no uncertain terms, you are ready to get married. Ask him what his five-year plan is and if marriage to you is part of his agenda. This kind of discussion is necessary to open up communication about his intentions. Most Black men have very specific ideas about marriage. All you have to do is ask him what they are.

If he is from a broken home, he probably believes fundamentally that marriage doesn't work. This may be an insurmountable stumbling block. If you help him cultivate friendships with happily married Black couples, he will see that in marriage you get out exactly what you put in, and that not all marriages have to end up like his parents'. If he comes to this realization, you two may have a chance.

By introducing him to other happily married Black men you increase the chances of his seeing that men can express themselves freely, openly, and lovingly without losing their macho status. Show and tell him that it's not corny or old-fashioned to want to be loved and adored. All human beings need to be loved and needed. Especially Black men!

Maybe he has a reputation of being "footloose and fancy free" but swears that he is ready to "settle down." Don't believe him unless he has actually demonstrated behavior that backs up his words. If he's acting like a "ladies man" looking for a wild time and is unable to get serious, simply acknowledge his behavior and move on to the next guy. Until he actually starts *acting* like a husband, he isn't ready to become one. No amount of schooling or cajoling will tame him if he is unwilling. Only *he* can control his behavior by consistently acting mature and responsible. Sooner or later his behavior will show you just how serious he is . . . or will be in the near future. *Pay attention!* The sooner you acknowledge exactly where he's coming from, the sooner you'll know if he's the right man for you.

Maybe *you* have established a wild and crazy image as a single woman, and now that you have decided you are ready to "settle down," he may not believe that you are capable of this mature behavior. In this case you will have to demonstrate through your actions and behavior (not just words) that you have already settled down (or are willing to). If he still doesn't believe you, give up on him. You'll just have to move on to someone who will take you seriously, someone who doesn't know any of your past behavior. You may have to find someone new who won't hold your past against you.

Another reason a guy acts like a fugitive has to do with his social and economic status. He doesn't feel that he would make a good enough provider. He wants to lay the world at your feet, but he knows he can't. So he doesn't even try and keeps running away. He sees you handling yourself with style and grace, so he feels threatened. He might feel that he is financially inadequate because you have a better job, more income, or greater economic potential. You may find that if he can't treat you like you deserve, he may treat you below par. This is unacceptable.

We encourage you to accept Brothahs who may not be wealthy, but who are making an honest attempt at surviving. However, you do not have to put up with complete financial ineptitude. There are Brothahs out there who have figured out how to make a way for themselves. Do not tolerate financial irresponsibility. Ever hear the saying "I can do bad all by myself"? You don't need to attach yourself to someone who cannot figure out how to make ends meet.

Look instead for a Black man who has a steady income, no matter how meager. Perhaps you can help him brainstorm how to parlay his steady but meager employment into something a little more financially rewarding. Sometimes all it takes is a great idea and a womban standing behind him with encouragement to create that second income that will help propel him on to the next tier of financial success. Or he might be willing to throw some brains and brawn into a project or business that the two of you can build together. *Beware* of the Brothah who pays lip service to your endeavor but really sabotages your budding growth by making you seem incompetent or who plans to help you, but doesn't. My (Cassandra's) husband used to come over to our tee-shirt workshop to iron and print up labels in his beautiful hand. He brought bags of rice, substantial gifts of food to feed the employees and the kids. That's also what is meant by support. Both tangible and intangible things.

You might be faced with an inequity in economic status. Many Black womben earn more than their mates. If this honestly doesn't bother you, then let him know. He may like you a lot, but may assume you'll dismiss him as a serious contender because of his economic status. Since Black womben have made such great strides in the work force, our levels of expectation are much higher than in years gone by. Black men are intimidated by these new expectations. They believe they have to measure up to our successes by matching our financial status. They think we believe the days of working together to get ahead in this life are over. Let your Black man know that you are willing to wait for material gains as long as he is making an honest attempt at bringin' home the bacon.

So what if you make and *save* more money than he does? No

one has to know your personal financial business but the two of you. Black men need the opportunity to get ahead. This does not mean, however, that you have to put up with nonsense. You should be able to tell the difference between a "jive" lazy fool and someone who's been out there working for "the man" with no opportunities in sight. Pool your resources and find a way to make it work. That's what our grandparents did. Look how far it got them.

Note: I, Monique, paid two hundred dollars for a weekend seminar at the Wharton Business School only to find out advice my grandparents had already told me for free. The advice was: The first most sound financial step you can take for the security of your future is to

Discipline yourself to save money on even the most modest salary!
Pay yourself while you're paying those bills.
You worked hard for your money. Bill yourself for your own
services.

He's Not Your Type . . . If He Acts like One of the Young Boyz

He may be shy and immature when it comes to serious relationships. Unless you are willing to spend many patient months, maybe even years, as he matures, you should consider leaving him alone and moving on to someone who is emotionally ready to meet you on your own terms.

He may have been "dogged" by an old girlfriend and may (unwittingly) be out for revenge. If he constantly makes blanket statements about the unacceptable traits of the entire female population or sneers at other womben who appear to be independent and self-sufficient, *beware*. He might just have an ax to grind and you don't want to be the cutting stone. Look for someone who basically accepts womben's independence and maturity and appreciates that such womben choose to be with men, despite the differences between them.

If he's commitment phobic as well, he just strings womben along until he feels it's getting too "close for comfort." This behavior is hard to spot right away. The only thing that might tip you off is if you casually bring up the topic of marriage and he freaks out immediately. Beware of this type of behavior, 'cause they usually hang in there for quite some time. Don't let him keep you on the hook for too long. We say *if he hasn't agreed to marry you after two years—DUMP HIM!* Look for someone who is willing to get married, to you, relatively soon.

You Know You've Got the Right One, Baby!!!

There are several kinds of positive behavior patterns men can exhibit that should clue you in to go after them. These Brothahs will exhibit great behaviors almost from the very beginning— that's one reason why they're so desirable. If he is behaving toward you like any one (or a combination) of *A Handy Man, A Dreamboat, A Black Butterfly,* then go for him in a *big* way, 'cause he is your new "type"!

You should realize that when Black men do kind, caring, and thoughtful things, it is their way of letting you know that they just might be "The One."

If he shows interest in you; in your life; in your thoughts; why isn't he your "type"?

_____

_____

_____

_____

He Is Your Type . . . If He Acts like a Handy Man

He's always there just when you need him. If he assures you that you've picked the perfect dress to wear to your presentation because it flatters your figure, he's your handy man. You hardly ever have to actually *ask* for his assistance 'cause he knows what you need before you do . . . usually. The sink's not leaking anymore. The light fixture in the linen closet works again. Things are running like clockwork, 'cause he's been there to fix all that needs fixing.

Your back isn't aching as much because he carries the groceries up five stories. Hot dinner is ready after a grueling day. The thank you notes were mailed in a respectable amount of time. Your father's birthday present was ordered from that catalog to arrive on time. Whatever the problem is, he takes the time to listen and help you figure out a solution. You can depend on his assistance in all aspects of your life. If he is trying to help you balance all of the drudgery that is the basis of your (anyone's) life, then he is *your* handy man.

He can be fair to gook-looking, but he doesn't usually try to be one of the "Pretty Boyz." He wears sports clothes that are always clean and unpretentious. In fact, you may struggle to get him into fancier *rags* (until you help him jazz up his wardrobe).

You can tell when a man is acting like a Handy Man, 'cause he *shows* that he cares about you in the most basic ways. He *likes* to do caring things in a very simple way. You may not get flowers *(maybe* on *special* occasions), but every other weekend you'll get to the grocery store in a clean car that runs like a charm. You will learn to depend on his reliability rather than his romanticism—and you may think that romance is not as wonderful when the mortgage payment and car insurance are due!

He Is Your Type . . . If He Acts like a Black Butterfly

Now if you don't care about *who* pays the bills (keeping in mind that it might usually be *you),* then the characteristics of a *Black Butterfly* won't faze you in the least. Talk about romance! He will wine you and dine you, give you candlelit baths, surround you with bubbles, cool you with dry wine. His artistic flair will enhance every encounter. This Brothah operates from his heart. He's what is known as a "feel-think" guy: His feelings influence his thinking. Other Brothahs can intellectualize with you forever, but this Brothah tells you what he's feeling, right from the start.

He'll drop you off at the station every morning and pick you up at your job every night, except when he's gigging, or working on a project with a serious deadline. But he'll always make it up to you. He'll keep the kitchen clean, the fridge well stocked with gourmet items and plenty of veggies and fruit, to help maintain your girlish figure. He may bring you one rose or pick a bouquet of garden flowers on his way home (even if they are from some-one else's garden).

If you love children, then a Black Butterfly is ideal. Children love his childlike, magical charm and appeal. He'll carry his own baby around endlessly. If the child can walk you'd never know it, 'cause it's feet will never touch the ground. He will shower love on both your child and you, as long as you appreciate him and his gifts. In other words, this man is a wonderful, inspiring man who will be a loving, caring partner. He just lives in an artistic world of his own.

You'll get all your phone messages, even the one from your old lover from your college days who is passing through town for the weekend. The Black Butterfly will encourage you to meet the Brothah for drinks—he's that secure in his love for you and you for him (of course you reciprocate). He'll try to figure out what it is that will make you happy and then try to provide it for you . . . even if it means getting a steady job for a few months. Not that he's not a hard worker, he's just not temperamentally suited for the traditional nine to five. As long as that doesn't bother you, it won't bother him.

Another way to recognize a Black Butterfly as he goes flitting through your life is to notice his circle of friends. Black Butter-flies usually have quite an eclectic assortment of people to hang out with. You'll find yourself surrounded by various creative and flamboyant personalities. These people can be intense, and they usually suggest unique and different things for you both to join in on: theatre openings, movie screenings, TV`show tapings, art openings, book signings, etc.

Special note: Sometimes his friends are more interesting than he is. You might get drawn into hanging out with him because you like the people he knows and the things he does. This is OK. Just make sure that it's *him* that you're drawn to and not his *lifestyle*.

His friends are just as important to him as you are, but for different reasons. They are usually engaged in all sorts of creative endeavors that require his intense involvement. As a musician, actor, dancer, writer, singer, comedian, or visual artist, he needs these associations to survive, so you must be prepared to share him with these friends. He, in turn, should be able to balance time spent with you and time spent creating or working on artistic projects. Don't allow jealousy of his exciting career to throw you. Although it may appear to be glamorous on the surface, you'll soon learn that his career requires just as much hard work and tenacity as yours does (assuming you're not in the arts yourself).

If you can peaceably share your life with him, accepting his pursuit of creative dreams as vital to his existence while at the same time acknowledging that these dreams may never materialize, then you will have a devoted partner with whom to look forward to a lifetime of love and beauty.

He Is Your Type . . . If He Acts like a Dreamboat

Romance is his middle name. He makes you feel like a queen. Dreamboats are always sweethearts. He really believes that you're *phat*, not fat! Dreamboats know how to compliment you without making you feel self-conscious. Just the sound of his sexy voice soothes you right when you need his help to keep your life sailing smoothly. The Dreamboat is usually quite handsome and an impressive dresser. This man will work long hours, but he'll definitely schedule in playtime. He may be distant at times, but he insists on a certain closeness with the womban he decides to make his wife.

You may find yourself with a bouquet of roses on your birthday, or one Friday he may pick up tickets for that boat ride or dance you'd been thinking about attending. Can't get a babysitter? Not to worry. He'll give the tickets to his brother or your sister, picking up a couple of videos on his way back to your place. After the kids are settled, he has time to talk to you about his goals and dreams to see how they compare with yours. He's a good listener too.

Caution: Because he is so *dreamy,* lots of times the Dreamboat doesn't trust womben because he's been tricked so many times. This may present a problem when it comes to his readiness quotient. If you've been dating him for years (five plus), he is probably marriage shy.

Sitting around your house with you is not a problem for this guy. He'll always bring something when he comes, because he's solid. It's incredible how clean this guy is. Imagine: a clean bathroom with a man in the house!?! . . . Heavenly, no? He wants to know what you think about his ability to beat his best buddy in chess. This kind of Brothah has a lot of knowledge that he's not ashamed to share. Even though he may not have finished college, his Motherwit combined with book learning (my Brothah *reads)* stimulates endless conversations and provides areas of mutual interest. A Dreamboat encompasses many of the characteristics of a smooth talker. He's romantic, but he's no Don Juan!

This Brothah may not sail you across the ocean on a luxury liner, and you probably won't be cruising the Bahamas in that sleek yacht either; but if your Dreamboat has a nice cabin that sleeps five or so and comes home to port every night, we'd call that Smooth Sailin'!

So you see, from now on *you have no "type"!* You simply date men who exhibit the kind of behavior and traits toward *you* that you now know to be desirable in a potential mate. Not what your mother or your friends know, but what *you* know. It's always nice if your family and friends think the guy is great, but it's *you* who knows what you want and need. They just *think* they know what's best for you. Remember, it's your life, and you have to take responsibility for living it. So *please,* please yourself. Either the folks will come around or they won't. When they see how happy you are, they'll start to wonder if *they're* wrong!

Since you now have no "type" or have determined that the right Black man can be your new "type," it's time to focus that energy and send it out into the Universe—so that you can draw him to you.

Your Pink Bubble Man

We now want you to meditate about your perfect man. Get into a quiet, relaxed state. Light a candle (pink for love or white for purity) if you have one. Imagine your ideal man. According to the "Heart Flower" meditation by Shakti Gawain, as found in her book *Creative Visualization* (see pp. 38–39), you should take all the best parts of old lovers—personality, looks, body build, color of eyes, hair type, clothes etc. Try to make this ideal man as real as possible. Visualize him walking around in clothes—business, play, pajamas. See him cooking you dinner, taking a bath, paying his bills. What qualities are you looking for in a man? What's his emotional makeup? What does his home look like? What's his occupation? Try and think of *everything,* even how he is in bed. Then meditate about this perfect fellow for about half an hour. Even if you have someone that you want to marry in mind, just use the best parts of him. After all, if he was "The One," you'd be married by now! Put your image of this ideal man into a pink bubble, since pink is the color of love. Take your time. Then release the pink bubble into the Universe. Imagine the bubble floating into the infinity of the Universe.

Don't worry if you're not successful at first. Pick another quiet time and place and try again. Once you've released your pink bubble into the Universe, *don't think about it ever again*. Gawain says that it will take about two years for the bubble to search the Universe, find the energy of your Pink Bubble Man, and bring it back to you. Two years may seem like a long time to wait, but if you're filling that time with increased growth, self-knowledge, and a few hundred dates, it will fly by!

By now, you should have released your "pink bubble" into the universe. You've let go of the intensity involved in finding a mate and are just having fun because you know that your positive energy—your pink glow—is going to bring your Black man into your sphere. You must be prepared to accept that he may not be the "type" of man you've always dreamed about. . . . He might be even better!

Jungle Fever

If you're not Black yourself, you still must determine if he's your type. You have to weigh the same factors about whom you want to spend the rest of your life with—plus you have a few added considerations.

If you suppose that you know everything there is to know about Black life . . . you still must consider a few very important things about interracial marriage. It ain't easy, no matter how you slice it. You will have to confront *anger* stemming from ancient prejudices—maybe regularly. If you are from a cosmopolitan center on the East or West Coast, you may adjust more easily because these places naturally encourage the coexistence of different cultures. Even if you've managed to work everything out, your families may discover various and sundry reasons why your relationship shouldn't work. Unfamiliar situations will test your levels of comfort and tolerance. Are you prepared to face these kinds of challenges throughout the rest of your life?

You can make the most of racial and cultural differences by sharing the best of both worlds. An emphasis on focusing only on the best pays off when children bless the union. Because interracial unions *must* include an acknowledgment and acceptance of the *permanent* differences that will remain an integral part of the partnership, they inherently encourage loyalty, fidelity, and compromise by all parties involved with the immediate family. A significant, conscious decision to cultivate an ongoing, ever-growing, and changing biracial marriage supports itself by highlighting diversity from the get-go.

Are you prepared to face these kinds of challenges throughout the rest of your life?　　　　　**Y　N**

How?

_____

_____

_____

You will encounter resentment from Sistahs who will feel that you are limiting their choice of eligible husbands . . . but guess what? Love knows no color. They're just gonna have to get over it, 'cause life is unpredictable and only you know in your heart what is right for you. As long as you are prepared to deal with reality, and not some romanticized view of what marriage to a Black man *might* be like, you'll be fine.

Name five positive benefits you can see coming from this interracial marriage.

_____

_____

_____

_____

_____

Name five negative aspects you can see to this marriage.

_____

_____

_____

_____

_____

By far the most disturbing and common result of interracial marriage is the total alienation of one side of the family because they choose not or are unable to tolerate the validity of the union.

If you are willing to walk away from your entire childhood and parental nurturing, ask yourself: Why is it so easy for me to detach myself from the most important relationships in my life to date?

_____

_____

_____

If you can detach so easily from this "birthright," what makes your marriage different that it won't end in a similar disconnection?

_____

_____

_____

Class Distinction

One of the most efficient ways of creating a smooth transition period for an interracial hook-up is to address not only racial issues but also class distinctions. We've noticed that in many cases, class differences between the two families contribute to many problems in interracial marriages. Because the race differences have such a profound impact on the meshing of the two cultures, sometimes class distinctions are simply overlooked.

There is the distinct possibility that either the bride or the groom is "marrying up." The accoutrements of the higher class may camouflage some personality traits you would never tolerate in someone of your own class and race. By the same token, a womban of another race who would normally never consider marriage with a Brothah just might *if* he is also offering a step up into a higher class.

We have noticed several potential brides and grooms who attributed differences solely to race were totally unaware that class was a factor. If you recognize that class as well as racial differences are in operation, you'll have a much better chance of making a mature and sound decision about interracial marriage.

Are you and your intended groom of different races and
the same class?   **Y N**

If you answered "No," will the class difference cause a significant
problem?   **Y N**

Why or why not?

_____

_____

_____

_____

Describe how you will balance the racial issues with the class issues.

_____

_____

_____

_____

Children of the Rainbow

The children of an interracial union must be treated with extra TLC. As the child of a white mother and a Black father, I, Monique, firmly believe that you will protect your children best by preparing them for the inevitable racism that, unfortunately, is out there waiting for them.

Even though you will create a hate-free environment for your children to flourish in, you must anticipate the worst they may encounter when dealing with the harsh, cruel world. You first must explain to them the basic fact that they will be hated for no other reason than the color of their skin. Make it clear that it's not in any way their fault and that, as their mother, you too will be hated, sometimes even more, because you love their father and gave birth to them. Words will _always_ hurt no matter how hard you try to protect your children from them. Just do your best to prepare them so that at least they won't be surprised in addition to being victims of prejudice.

We encourage you to involve your children in activities and friendships that bolster pride in both sides of their cultural background. Raising Black children, especially Black boys, is definitely not an easy labor of love these days. We advise that you carefully consider exactly how hard it may be and decide if you're up to the challenge.

Do you think you can meet *all* the challenges inherent in
  raising Black children?   **Y N**

If you answered "No," think twice before you go for some more of that brown sugar. If you answered "Yes," more power to you. We're all Sistahs under the skin. As long as you can deal with the wrath of ignorant, small-minded people, you can have a happy marriage.

Now that you have explored all the possibilities as to who your husband might end up being, imagine finding him in the perfect situation. Haven't a clue where to look? Try at least three of our Six Trix, guaranteed to get you closer than you've ever been before.

Long-Distance Love

If you do meet someone, and he lives five hundred miles away, don't be so quick to dismiss the idea of getting involved. There are many advantages to long-distance relationships, including so-called commuter marriages.

If you are used to living alone and ordering your life to suit only yourself, having a husband who lives away from you on a part-time basis allows you to couple the freedom of your single days with the intimacy of a beloved partner. Living apart but being married combines the two. This joining takes dedication, devotion, and maturity. It is not a good idea for one who is or has a tendency to become jealous. It also requires an independent, faithful man and womban.

Have you met a potential mate who lives far away?   **Y N**

Do you engage in many social activities alone?   **Y N**

Do you have a good job with good benefits?   **Y N**

You want to be married, but you don't want to relocate. While on vacation in the Bahamas, you meet a man who fulfills your every fantasy of a Dreamboat . . . but he lives in Boston and you live in Cleveland! He has finally proposed marriage to you and you have accepted. Now he wants to know when you are moving to Boston. He's considered Cleveland, but decided to remain where he is. Each of you has a job you care about, in a town with a comfortable network of friends and family. You're both in your forties and have been through the wringer a few times. You really love each other but can't see how either of you can relocate, especially since you've both started accumulating equity and accomplishing some material goals. You see the partner of your autumn years slipping down the garden path, away from you, leaving you lonely and alone.

But wait. There's an alternative to this scenario. You could marry, visit each other periodically, and take an early retirement, mutually deciding where to live during the retirement years. Although it's now a media fad, commuter marriages have been in existence in the Black community for hundreds of years.

Have you ever had a long-distance relationship?   **Y N**

Are you jealous?   **Y N**

Do you like to travel?   **Y N**

Musicians have always lived away from their homes, sometimes for many years at a time, yet still managed to have wives and children. Since the great West Indian migration to the United States in the 1940s and '50s, many West Indian families have thrived with one spouse living and working in the States and one spouse living and working in the islands.

A long-distance relationship requires much patience and self-sufficience. Most people who are able to carry this off have usually experienced at least one long-distance relationship before, perhaps while away at college. Most of the time these relationships don't work out simply because the partners are not really mature enough to handle the many stresses that are involved. You must be very clear about what you need and want out of a relationship.

Over the last two years, Elmer and I have entered into just such a relationship. After his mother's seventy-fifth birthday, he remained on Curaçao, the island of his birth, while I and my school-aged son returned to the States. Elmer has been working and helping his mother and family there ever since. The traveling distance is so great that we've only been able to see each other once or twice a year, but the separation has allowed us to focus on individual needs and personal-growth issues that would have been almost impossible to do had we been living together. It is difficult at times, but, so far, the positives have outweighed the negatives.

There are, however, many tough circumstances that accompany this choice. You will miss many small, trivial events in addition to the momentous occurrences that bind a couple together, from acquiring the first big sales commission to signing the contracts for a new deal. Some of these things can be compensated for with phone calls and surprise visits, but there will be times when you question the wisdom of your decision to live apart.

Do you have a good support system in place?   **Y N**

Are you an effective communicator?   **Y N**

Are you a good letter writer?   **Y N**

Incredible communication skills are required to implement and maintain this kind of relationship. You not only have to give "good phone," but you also have to be on top of letter writing and mailing small packages. Books, music, cards, and letters must continually cross each other in the mail. Awaiting that special card or letter from your sweetheart can be one of the most passionate times of your life . . . And speaking of passionate, you don't have to worry about getting tired of each other sexually if you only see each other once or twice every few months. The problem will more likely be getting out of bed long enough to take care of other business and see friends and family.

Fidelity is also an issue with long-distance lovers. There are the traditional definitions of fidelity and then there are the individual definitions of fidelity. As long as your perceptions and beliefs about it are the same or are able to be "mapped" onto each other's with plenty of open, honest communication, this issue can be dealt with without too much heartache and hurt feelings.

What is your definition of fidelity? _____

_____

_____

_____

Do you and your partner agree on this definition?   **Y N**

If not, how do your interpretations differ? _____

_____

_____

Sometimes in these relationships one partner gets tired of traveling so much and will decide to take the plunge and relocate. All the better. This way you two are able to leisurely plan the relocation—with time to shift support systems and employment.

Long distance lovers must be well-versed in the fine art of negotiation. Each person must be flexible and have a good sense of humor. If you have most of these qualities (and a prospect), then you will probably be able to make a long-distance love work for you.

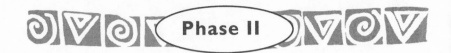

GeTTin' A bRoThAh
To NoTiCe THe
nEw YoU

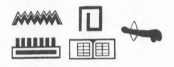

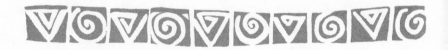

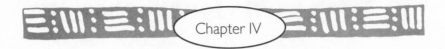
SIX TRIX

> ## *Word from the Brothahs*
>
> **Do you think that there is a lack of places to meet Black men?**
>
> "I'm not saying go to a club to meet people but you can meet 'em anywhere."
>
> "I never met anyone in a club—except my wife!"
>
> "I met my wife in a club. She was there with a friend of ours. A friend of mine introduced us."
>
> **How would you advise a womban to get a date with you?**
>
> "Call me up."

We've come up with what we think are six surefire methods of meeting Black men. Use them all over and over again until you meet "The One."

Note: Don't worry that there are not loads of available men in your area. You only need one to marry!

Trick #1: Go for the Glow

Volunteer to *pass out flyers* for an organization you've joined, a club you've formed, or an event you feel strongly about (such as Maya Angelou or Farrakhan speaking). While standing and passing out flyers at events, you can spot interesting men and approach them on the street or anywhere. You have an excuse to speak to someone you may not have had the guts to talk to before. People notice you and get a chance to check you out. Make sure you look your best on the day of the event, 'cause you never know if he came to check out Maya Angelou— or you! Many charitable organizations or fledgling artists' organizations would be grateful for the opportunity to make their work known to a wider audience. You will be giving off good vibes as a result of your deed and will attract people with positive energy.

Trick #2: Rock the Jock's Socks

Attend sports events, like marathon road races, softball games, especially basketball games. Pick a sport that you enjoy or that genuinely interests you (once you get the guy, though, you have to maintain your level of interest). Integrity is important in any endeavor. One friend chose basketball because she is nearly six feet tall. She went after the players in the "Elderly League," former NBA and international players, the youngest of whom was about twenty-nine. There are lots of different types of men there. Make sure that you have plenty of flyers to hand out or business or social cards (a social card is simply your name and home number if you can't field calls at work).

Note: Remember, men go to games to get away from their womben (wives, girlfriends, mothers-in-law, mothers, daughters). So while cheering those Knicks or Bullets, if a fine Brothah catches your eye, just discreetly slip him a card, fade into the crowd, and let him enjoy the game with his boyz.

Trick #3: Wait to Wait

Another thing that you can do at one of these large events is to choose your spot when you get in line for refreshments, souvenirs, etc. Wait until you see an attractive guy get on line and then get on line behind him. While you're waiting, you can strike up a conversation, which always unfolds naturally in such a situation. Always carry your cards, flyers, and a pen. Have a "little red book" handy for all those red-hot numbers, and you'll be all set. This trick works not just at sporting or social events but also at the Department of Motor Vehicles, Ticketron outlets, your local utilities office, etc.

Trick #4: Classified Ad-venture

Place an ad! Many of you may scoff at this idea, because it's corny or scary, but believe us, *it works!* One womban placed a free ad in the *Village Voice* person-to-person handout. She had twenty-eight dates in thirty days! We recommend screening before seeing, but if you're bored, what the heck! Make sure the ad

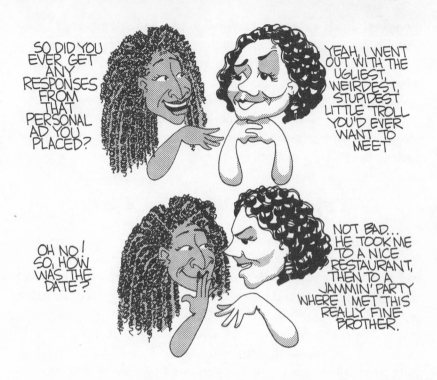

says a couple of things unique to you and your quest. Get help from a friend to make it succinct, snappy, and successful. A few Black magazines accept ads, or you can place one in an upscale local weekly magazine or the local newspaper. The newspaper will guarantee quantity, the magazine will ensure quality. Placing an ad in a magazine will probably be costly, but the respondent will more than likely be a person with some disposable income.

Once you've picked out a guy to respond to, get together with a few of your single girlfriends who have also placed ads and plan a *singles' soiree*. Invite the victims (we mean dates), to a local family-style restaurant (preferably one with dancing) or to an upscale bar/restaurant with dancing. More likely than not, somebody will come out of the evening with a likely prospect. Three to five couples allow for great mingling (just hope that all of you don't go for the same guy—at least not at the same time!).

At least twice a year, *Ebony* magazine has a feature article called "Most Eligible Bachelors/Bachelorettes." Black singles who want to meet other Black singles write in (enclosing a photo) and ask to be featured. Many of them are selected and subsequently receive letters from men and womben who want to meet them. You can either submit yourself to be featured as a Bachelorette or write to one of the eligible Bachelors in care of the magazine.

Trick #5: Use the Internet to Catch Your Fly Guy

In this age of the information highway, it may be easier to meet a compatible person *online*. Networks such as America Online, Prodigy, and CompuServe are a few of the national computer networks where you can converse with numerous people. You can acquire the software for free from computer magazines like *PC World* or *MAC World* or in the mail. You usually get ten free hours of online time, so you can see if you enjoy *surfin' the net*. Once you log on, don't be afraid to bring up race, since you *are* looking for a Black man. Check out NetNoir on America Online. Or you can enter "rooms" that are designated Black, like the Ebony Room. Many users already know each other, but don't let that discourage you. You can always send an "IM" (an immediate/instant message) to someone by e-mail so he can speak to you privately. It's amazing what crazy things Brothahs and Sistahs will say while surfing the net. It gives you the perfect opportunity to exercise the most obscure parts of your imagination. You can flirt, meet people of all ethnic types, philosophies, and sexual orientations. You choose a cool alias or abbreviate your real name for identification. The alias is helpful especially if you go into one of the kinky or sex "rooms." (Sex rooms are the ultimate adventure for exploring your erotic fantasies. Talk about *safer sex!*)

If you really want to meet someone, just start talking straight from the heart. You never know, sometimes people monitor conversations without ever speaking. A great guy may be online, want to interact or communicate with you after realizing a real interest, and decide to send an IM. His IM will appear on your screen, and you can then respond or not. You can pull up and check out the person's profile before you respond. If the rooms you're interested in are full (the Ebony Room is often full), you can create your own room to discuss a topic that is important or interesting to you.

There are lots of abbreviations that people use to speak to each other during chat sessions using e-mail. Have fun making up some of your own. Here are some frequently used codes:

{{name}}:	Hugging the person named.
BCNU:	Be seein' you.
BTW:	By the way.
FWIW:	For what it's worth.
IANAL/D:	I am not a lawyer/doctor.
IMHO:	In my humble opinion.
LOL:	Laughing out loud.
OIC:	Oh, I see.
OL:	Out loud

ROTFL: Rolling on the floor laughing.
RUMRF: Are you male or female?

Don't be afraid to go surfin' on the Internet. Just watch out for the crazies!

Trick #6: Bounty Hunters

Trick #6 is the pièce de résistance.

bounty hunter n. 1. one who hunts predatory or wild animals or criminals and outlaws for a reward, inducement, or payment.

We've heard about womben who offer rewards to their families, friends, and co-workers to find them a mate. The idea is that whoever introduces her to the guy she eventually marries wins the prize. This gives your family and friends incentive to come up with quality dates—that is, men who at least remotely resemble your Pink Bubble Man. Since you've made such a detailed image of your Pink Bubble Man, you will easily be able to describe your man to your Bounty Hunters.

One womban offered a round-trip ticket to Puerto Rico from New York City or Atlanta. You could offer a trip to the Bahamas, Mexico, Montreal, wherever, depending on your point of departure. Other ideas for prizes are a weekend for two at a four-star hotel of your choice; tickets to a Broadway show; dinner for two at a five-star restaurant; a massage or facial; a nice piece of jewelry, etc. (Make sure that the prize will be sufficiently motivating to your family and friends!)

Of course, the prize depends on your financial means, but just add it to your wedding budget. If you *really* can't afford a substantial prize, then offer to do a dirty or unpleasant job for an extended period of time, such as free babysitting one weekend a month for six months; weekly housecleaning for six months to a year; washing and cleaning the car for six months to a year . . . catch the drift? It's got to be *major.*

We've culled a list of places to meet men. Add these to some of the trix we've given (and that you've discovered over the years) for greater effectiveness.

Reminder: Always carry a pen so you can easily give and take numbers!

Sports Bars, Cafés, Coffeehouses, and Restaurants: Armed with your cards, flyers, and little red book, you don't have to be a wallflower anymore!

Book and Record Stores: These places are just made for browsing. You can always strike up a conversation about whatever section you're in. The Barnes and Noble's and Borders bookstores in most major cities have coffee shops. These kinds of places are becoming notorious as pick-up spots, so be aware.

Supermarkets and Laundromats: We all eat and get our clothes dirty. Most of us don't have personal shoppers, maids, or valets. Our research has shown that people who end up marrying usually resided within a three-mile radius of each other, so *shop locally!* You may find better bargains elsewhere, but just think of the extra expenditures as investment funds.

Houses of Worship: If you have a strong religious background, churches, mosques, and the like are "inspirational" places to meet men, and not only at the main service. Don't rule out the social groups or special-interest groups that are an integral part of these organizations. Pick one or two—check out a couple of meetings for prospects and decide which group to join. The young male mentoring programs are a good choice. You can offer to be a sort of "den mother" to the fellas. Just because it's a program for men doesn't mean that you can't help.

Concerts and Political and Cultural Events: Like sporting events, these offer a large selection of people, long lines, and a common interest. Again, arm yourself with flyers and social or business cards. Don't forget your little red book!

Weddings and the Workplace. Once you've informed your Bounty Hunters, these places become gold mines, especially big weddings and large commercial establishments. At work, try not to date someone in your department so that if it doesn't work out, you don't have to see each other every day.

Museums and Exhibits: Check out the listings in local magazines and newspapers for African, Caribbean, South American, and African American/Canadian museums and exhibits. Many of our positive Brothahs are race-proud. They support and are influenced by our cultural art and artifacts. These places also offer intimate crowds and provide the perfect setting for great conversations.

Note: If you can, get invited or purchase tickets to exhibit openings. People are there to socialize as well as to view. You, of course, will have your weapons on hand (cards, little red book, flyers, etc.).

Small Theater and Dance Performances: In addition to support-ing our own artists and culture, these events usually have small audi-ences. The opportunity for single people to meet and mingle abound, especially during intermission and just after the performance.

Hint: Use a line like "If you liked this performance, you'll love this event . . ." (and hand over a flyer).

The Malls and Department Stores: Especially check out men's stores and men's departments. While shopping for a gift for your "brother," "father," "uncle," or "son," you can approach a hot prospect for advice or an opinion. (So what if Dad's birthday isn't for four months?!)

The Great Outdoors: People are creatures of habit. Like shopping and doing the laundry, they usually bike, jog, or walk the same route at the same time every day. Since you are exercising to keep your body healthy, just vary your schedule or route. You'll see many more differ-ent men than usual. We counseled one friend to learn how to fall off her bike (by pretending to hit a rock or something) without hurting herself, so that when she saw a guy she liked she could literally throw herself at his feet. (She was still practicing as we went to press!)

Professional and Social Organizations: When you belong to or join a professional or social organization, your chances of meeting a potential mate are greatly enhanced. There are many organizations to choose from—church organizations, 100 Black Women, 100 Black Men, Links, or one of the various groups of business, professional, or political men and womben in your area. The list goes on and on. Find one that suits your interests and lifestyle. Regular meetings and functions provide great opportunities to meet Black men.

Jack and Jill of America, Inc.: Although this group is family-oriented, it's a good place for single parents to meet each other. Not only does it provide a social network for your children, but it also widens your field of potential Bounty Hunters.

House Parties: This is almost as good as being introduced to a man by a friend or family member. Usually you know who's throwing the jam, so you know the type of crowd. Black men like house parties 'cause they can really let loose and have a slammin' time! They are usually looking for single womben too!

Fraternity and Sorority Dances: These usually have a mixed-age crowd because many frats and sororities have graduate chapters. Expect to meet men of any age!

TV Talk Shows and Black Radio Programs: You'd be surprised at how many people tune in, see or hear someone they like, and then write in to the show and ask for a meeting with the person they're interested in. Tune in to your local radio station that has an urban/pop music format; from time to time it will sponser a dating promotion.

Don't forget: Never give your telephone number to a man who won't give you his. Don't accept office numbers. He probably has something to hide, like a wife or a live-in girlfriend!

All you really have to do to get a date is look good, feel good about yourself, and be receptive, aware, and in the right place at the right time.

Just putting yourself (a "together self") where men are will get you a date.

Caution: Don't worry if it seems that your "requirements" are not being fulfilled. Even the unappealing guys have friends. By dating outside your usual channels, you'll widen your circle of acquaintances, which in turn will increase the likelihood of meeting your mate.

Attention: Everywhere you go there is an opportunity to meet Black men! It's up to you.

Which trick(s) worked for you?

_____

_____

_____

_____

_____

Where did you find it easiest to meet Black men?

_____

_____

_____

Have you remembered to flirt with all of the Black men
  you've come in contact with in your daily life?   **Y N**

Warning: Don't let your first dates take place in a movie house. Yes, it gives you a topic to discuss, but you'll have wasted a couple of good hours in a noncommunicative situation.

You've gathered enough information from dating to know exactly what you need and want. We strongly advise husband hunting vigorously for six months, and then taking a break for a while. That's how I, Monique, met my husband Bobby. I was on Christmas vacation in the Virgin Islands, where an old college friend introduced us. I had decided to give husband hunting a break while I was away. I'd decided to let go and let God. I swear, all of that energy I had put into making myself ready paid off when I least expected it to! So get ready, get set, go . . .

Now that you know how to meet 'em, it's time to learn how to greet 'em! Ready!?!?

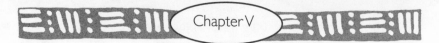
OpEnInG cLAMs

Word from the Brothahs

"I like aggressive womben because it sometimes takes the pressure off me."

When you first start dating, how can a womban tell if you're not interested in being in a serious relationship with her?

"I don't think men even know yet. We don't know. It has to escalate...gradually over time. She can't know right away and you can't know right away even if you're serious."

"When she wants to go out during the daytime...and you don't want to be seen with her."

"Early in the relationship a lot of men are good actors. They put on some good shows. We all know...we've done it."

"I mean, if the womban tells you what she wants, whether she's telling you the truth or not, at least it gives you something, somewhere to go. Most men, no matter how cool they act, don't have a clue. You see a womban over there, you don't know where to...start."

First and foremost; Always remember to *smile and say "Hello" to every Black man you see.*

We've found that if you ask any man a series of questions within the first five minutes of meeting him, he will tell you almost anything you want to know about himself. After that he clams up and won't tell you a thing. So make a practice of asking a man some basic questions as soon as you meet him. You never know, he may be "The One." Always ask *"Are you single?"* first. Men usually smile, then answer you directly. Whether they are free or not, they are flattered that you are interested in them at all. Asking personal questions is the fastest way to let any man know that you are interested in him. Since you just met him, he doesn't feel threatened or that he has anything to lose; so usually he'll tell the truth and give you an honest answer.

We realize this sounds a little pushy, but in the first five minutes he won't even know what hit him! Most men like the attention. Their egos love it! One girlfriend (now married) said her then "Perfect Stranger" used to say, "Boy, you certainly ask a lot of questions." But she swears that he answered all of her questions, much to her surprise. This way you find out if he is appropriate for you right away.

Be aware that many men, especially urban guys, are on to this. So you have to keep your questions to a minimum and be creative in the way you present them. Try to work your questions into the conversation in a flirtatious manner. Rapid-fire interrogation is definitely going to turn any man off. If you think that you might have problems with this aspect of the program, practice on some male friends until it has become somewhat natural for you to "interrogate" cleverly.

If he is available and you like him, don't hesitate to let him know it! Give him a big smile if he says he's single!

Then ask *"Do you have any children?"* Let him know if you have children too. Many men will not bring this up until they think they might want to get serious about you. But we feel you should know what the whole package is, right up front. If you don't want a ready-made family, isn't it better to know his situation in the first five minutes? And if you don't mind having children as part of the deal, at least you know what you're getting yourself into.

We suggest you ask *"Do you think you'll ever get married?"* next. Men are very logical human beings. We found that whatever he tells you his life plan is in those first five minutes will be exactly what he does. If he tells you that he's engaged to someone and is dating on the side "till that day," don't think that you can change his mind and get him to marry you instead. If he tells you, "I'm not the marrying kind," *believe* him. Don't think, "Oh I'll change him." If he tells you, "I want to wait until I'm forty-five," don't doubt him because . . .

Men do exactly what they say they are going to do!

On your first meeting, you can also ask a series of questions like *"What do you do?"* *"Where do you live?"* *"How old are you?"* *"What sign are you?"* and whatever else you might want to know. You *should not* ask question after question after question. That really turns men off and tips them off to the fact that you're on a "mission." Throughout the initial conversation don't ask more than two or three questions. If you've managed to hold his attention longer than the first few moments, continue to mix in the rest of your questions as they seem to naturally fit into the conversation. Ask questions about everything that is important to you, especially sex, politics, money, and religion, *but don't play 20 Questions*. Spread some of the more serious questions out over the next several dates.

Remember: Try not to reveal anything about yourself while you're obtaining all of this pertinent information about him. The less he knows about you, the better: He'll have to keep taking you out on dates to figure out who you are. You'll intrigue him by making him wonder..."Who is this self-assured womban who is so interested in me?"

What are some of the questions you would like to ask a prospective mate?

_____

_____

_____

_____

Here are some interviewing rules:

1. Direct the conversation to a specific topic.
2. Let him talk.
3. Show interest in and remember what he says.
4. Do not censor his comments.

5. Do not criticize or ridicule him.
6. Make sure he knows that you like him.
7. Do not waste time with someone you don't like.

If you realize right away that he is someone you don't like, see if he may have qualities that may help you meet other, more appropriate men. For example, let's say he's not for you because he's too good-looking and you can see he's a ladies' man, but in those first five minutes he tells you he works for a major record label and he's always looking for a womban to have as a friend to take to all those industry parties. You could go with him and maybe meet Mr. Right while you're just hangin' out.

So don't be afraid to open that clam as soon as you find it, because that may be the last chance you get until he's *ready* to tell you things.

Get Geared Up

Dress your best. Wear clothes that flatter your figure and bring out your coloring. Don't dress too provocatively unless you *know* for a fact that his last womban wore a 40DD, flaunted it all, and he loved it. However, this doesn't mean that you should be covered head to toe, unless you're Muslim! Otherwise, save the sexy stuff for the bedroom or for intimate dinners. We don't mean that you should change your whole wardrobe; just check out his taste and try to complement or contrast, tastefully. Try wearing only your best outfits. Reassess your wardrobe. Be as ruthless in your closet as you are in your manhunt. If you attract him only with your body, by wearing seductive clothing, how are you going to keep him with your mind? *You have to impress him with your personality.*

Food for Thought

Now that you've met him and he seems appropriate, here are some tips to keep him interested. Make sure he knows you like him by smiling a lot, telling him you think he's got beautiful eyes, etc.

What are some of the ways you indicate that you find someone attractive?

_____

_____

_____

Can you verbalize these ways and communicate them to a man?   **Y N**

If yes, what are some of the things you can say to a man to tell him that you are interested in him?

_____

Work on solving only one problem at a time. One of the initial problems you might be faced with may be his inability to reveal his inner feelings. Don't make a common mistake of playing the "cool chick" role. Don't be one of the "oh, so modern" womben who never presses that ladies' man into telling you how he really feels about you.

Playing it cool might be appropriate in the very beginning, but eventually it's wise to move toward establishing closeness and intimacy. Black men, like most men, find it extremely difficult to express how they feel emotionally. So, if you can coax him into trusting you enough to let his inner feelings show, you'll be well on your way to cultivating a lifelong mate.

Black men often associate a likely mate with a womban who can actually help them get in touch with their own feelings. Ask really personal questions about his life. Don't let him get off the hook without giving you a direct answer. If he starts to squirm, be persistent. This takes a great deal of finesse, but it's usually worth the time and effort. You have to have the guts to pull off this type of assertive approach or it won't work. We'll let you gals in on a secret: Make him feel good about himself, whenever you're around him. This will make it easier for him to fall in love with you. Though he may not consciously realize why, he'll find himself wanting to be around you. Hence, the opportunity to trap him with your charms.

We feel that when you are dating a man who isn't Mr. Right, it's important to tell him, in no uncertain terms, that you are seriously looking for a husband. He may be great and "all that," but he's not "The One." Inform him that you'd still like to date him, but let him know that he has to be prepared to let you go when you meet Mr. Right. By warning him, you take the pressure off the relationship.

Second, Black men love home cooking. So on your second or third date, offer to make a nice meal—lunch or dinner. The adage still holds true even in our rushed lifestyles, that "the way to a man's heart is through his stomach." Candlelight and soft music work wonders. One of the easiest man traps to set is to have a neat and tidy house or apartment every time he visits. He'll long to be back in your tranquil hideaway, where he is pampered and adored, away from his hectic bachelor life.

How often do you clean your place? _____

Thoroughly? _____

It's been said that men respond well when you ask them questions that their mother used to ask, questions like *"Are you hungry?" "Are you tired?"* etc. Black men don't get much respect from society at large, so you can help make them feel pampered with just a little TLC and attention.

Pay some attention to what Dr. Harville Hendrix teaches in his video series. He says the reason we nag our mates and expect them to cater to our every whim, without our telling them what our needs are, directly results from the first two learned experiences we had as newborn babes. Our omnipotent parents always knew exactly what we needed or wanted without our telling them; and crying in the loudest, nastiest "shrill" always got an immediate response.

This was our first experience of "love." So our unconscious thinks that "true love" involves someone who not only tolerates such behavior but seeks it out. We must retrain our unconscious memory to accept adult true love, which is considerate, patient, understanding, and forthright about needs and wants.

Communication is the key to building a relationship. Listening is the most important first step. You'd be surprised at what he might say if you just give him the chance. But try to make yourself hold back. Sometimes you may even need to bite your cheek. As we said earlier, in the beginning try to tell him as little about *yourself* as possible. Then he'll have to ask you on another date, so he can learn more about you (you sensitive, mysterious lady). Get the picture? Communicate, but don't reveal all your charms on the first date. (Or even on the second!)

Ten Telephone Tips

Tip #1: Don't buy into the old theory of never calling a guy. If you want to call him and you have something to communicate, by all means call the Brothah. Just don't allow yourself to babble. Keep the conversation short, sweet, and to the point.

Tip #2: Cultivate a telephone voice that sounds sultry and sexy when you're talking to that special man, and *please* say "Hello, this is...[*your name*]" when you call. Especially if he lives with other people. The more polite and friendly you are, the more likely your message will get through.

Tip #3: There's no safer sex than *phone sex!*

Tip #4: If a womban answers his phone, don't jump to conclusions about who she is. She could be a relative or close friend. Be polite and leave your name and a message. However, if the woman says "OK" with an attitude, make sure you get her name. Next time you see or talk to him, casually mention that you spoke to So-and-So the last time you called. Check his reaction or simply and innocently ask who she is.

Tip #5: Always be the first to end the conversation. (See rule number 1.)

Tip #6: Return his calls promptly, but *never* sit by the phone waiting.

Tip #7: Don't act jealous when his beeper goes off...even if you are! The best way to slay the Green-Eyed Monster is to never let it rear its ugly head!

Tip #8: Don't get frustrated if he has a job that prevents him from talking on the phone. He may have an extremely demanding position. Maybe personal phone calls aren't allowed. Or he may have limited access to the phone—whatever. Just chill and enjoy the occasions when you do speak with him by phone.

Tip #9: If he's always on the phone or constantly getting beeped, decide *now* if you can deal with this behavior, 'cause it ain't gonna change! It might even get worse as he becomes more successful.

Tip #10: Don't keep leaving messages on his answering machine. Leave one message and wait until he calls back. If he doesn't return your call promptly, wait until the next day and leave one more message.

Whether you're on the phone or "all the way live," there's always an opportunity to show how understanding and compassionate you are. But *do not give unsolicited advice!* Dr. John Gray assures us, in his book *Men Are from Mars and Women Are from Venus*, that men absolutely hate this! Try to let him do whatever he's doing his way. No mothering! And always try to say "Would you" instead of "Could you" when asking him to do anything for you. It may not make a difference to you, but it will make a big difference to him.

All of our advice should be tempered with common sense. You should do what you think the situation requires. For example, in one instance we say, "Ask questions that his mother asked him, so he'll associate you with a nurturing figure." Then here we say, "No mothering"—meaning nagging. What we mean is to adopt the positive traits of mothering, not the negative ones.

Even though you are taking an active role to find your husband, once you've met him and you think he might be "The One," back off some. Give him the space to be able to pursue you. No matter how dreamy he is, you must maintain an independent attitude until he suggests marriage!

Go for the Real Deal

Accept a Black man as he is. Do not idealize or romanticize him. Be able to live with who he is right now, because he may never reach his potential, sometimes through no fault of his own. This is a trap many of our Sistahs fall into. The deck is stacked against him, so act accordingly. Acceptance through empathy and understanding are the most effective ways to promote a constructive relationship. Accept that he is fighting against great odds and empathize that he may have a low self-esteem because of this. Embrace him as a Black man trying to do something positive with his life and realize that sometimes he may be having a hard time of it. If you can take him as he comes you'll be all right, Sis. But don't marry him with the notion that he will become too much more than he already is right now.

Many successful Black people struggle with subtle racism every single day. All you can do is do the best you can. Don't judge yourself by the "special" standards of excellence set for African Americans by the majority culture. Judge yourself by what you know to be universally true—set and satisfy your own standards of excellence. If he doesn't want to or (can't) live up to your standards, forget him and move on to a Black man who has not succumbed to the power of negative thinking. There are lots of positive Brothahs out there. Don't give up on the Black men who are making great strides in their lives despite the daily challenges they face.

We're not saying that Black men don't reach great heights, they do! It's just that if you meet a man in his late thirties to mid forties, he's not going to advance too much farther than he is right now, financially, emotionally, socially, etc.

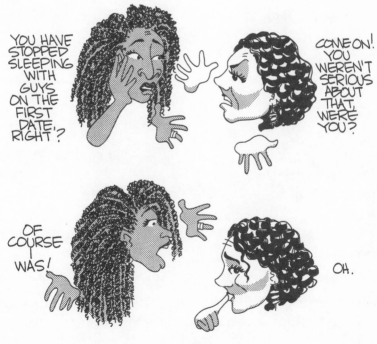

The Heavy Date(s)

We know that the wedding is still a remote possibility, but just think about it. After you've dated for a while, you may *think* you know each other. Forget it! You are still on your best behavior. Now it's time for a *heavy date*.

On heavy dates you bring up some of the questions you still have and the revelations you have uncovered during the initial getting-to-know-you period. Questions that deal with taboo topics—AIDS tests, sex, drugs, politics, religion—fit into this category.

From what you know so far, are his goals and values compatible with yours?

_____

_____

By now you know what religion, if any, he practices. Does it
jibe with your beliefs? **Y N**
Is he uncomfortable with your spirituality, or is he the live and
let live type? _____

Will his attitude change if he were ever to have kids? **Y N**

Remember: You're in this for the long haul, so any major differences may become insurmountable obstacles after the wedding!

You've hung out together enough to know which substances he abuses, be it nicotine, alcohol, "recreational" drugs, food, money, etc. How do you feel about it?

_____

_____

Let him know.

Smokers Beware

Be aware that a lot of men don't like it when womben smoke. If you have met someone who seems to be worthwhile and has expressed a sincere objection to your habit, we suggest you follow these tips to show your consideration for his feelings and health, especially if you don't expect to quit anytime soon.

Tip #1: Don't smoke on the street.

Tip #2: Don't set a bad example by smoking in front of children.

Tip #3: Don't smoke while he's eating.

Tip #4: Try not to smoke immediately after sex or meals.

Tip #5: If you must smoke around him, go to another room or outside.

Tip #6: Be aware of the smell of smoke that lingers in your clothes, hair, and living space.

Tip #7: Realize that down the line your smoking could become a major issue, causing him to think twice about marrying you.

Tip #8: Consider quitting. (Do what Iyanla van Zant advises: "Ask God to bless your lungs *every* time you take a puff." She explains that there's nothing we can do to *make* people quit until they are ready to quit themselves. There is some reason why they can't stop smoking at this time in their lives. We pray that you will find the conviction to quit. We know how hard it is 'cause Cassandra is still struggling with quitting herself.)

Do your politics jibe? **Y N**

You don't necessarily have to belong to the same party, but it helps if you have a similar ideology and depth of commitment.

These are all tough questions, but you should be able to ask him. If you are unable or unwilling to, your relationship may not be as advanced as you think or hope it is. If any of the questions seem to make him uncomfortable, that's OK—as long as he answers them! If he can't or won't, it may indicate that he will not be open to you and your needs in a long-term relationship. You may need to reevaluate the situation.

What questions have you avoided or haven't had the nerve to ask?

_____

_____

_____

What questions was he unwilling to answer?

_____

_____

_____

There is nothing more satisfying than to feel that someone has listened to everything you've said and understands and empathizes with you. So when you two have those heart-to-heart conversations, mirror back to him (summarize) what he's said to you. Then tell him how you feel about how he feels. He'll appreciate your compassion. (Hopefully, he'll empathize with you too. If he doesn't, then maybe he's not right for you, after all.)

Don't be afraid to make him laugh or to laugh about things he says or does. This goes for when you're in bed as well. I, Monique, told my husband that I will divorce him the day he stops making me laugh! Humor can help almost any situation. We realize it's impossible to teach someone how to have a great sense of humor. All we can say is . . . lighten up sometimes! Life is only as intense as you allow it to be.

Family Matters

We suggest that you meet his family early on. Even if his immediate family doesn't live close by, a sibling or cousin can also be a good gauge of his background and family ties. You'll be surprised at how much you'll learn about him from just one visit with his folks. It will also give you a chance to check out how he relates to people. Of course he'll relate to his family differently than to other people, but here is an excellent opportunity to hone your observation skills. This meeting may give you a good indication of just how compatible you are. He's made up of his familial experiences, right? So if you get along with them, most likely you'll get along with that part of him. Plus, in-laws play a huge role in marriage. So test the waters gently, and just be your naturally charming self.

Perhaps your intended is an orphan or is estranged from his family. You can still check out the extent of his family ties by the quality and quantity of his friendships. If he has at least one close friend, you can observe the depth and closeness of that relationship, as though it were familial. If he doesn't have at least one or two close friends (including platonic female friendships) or if he has tons of friends, none of whom he is close to, then beware. He might just be a loner or be new in town. But then again he might be antisocial, someone who just doesn't get along with other people. Unless this suits you just fine (and we mean for the *long* haul), take it slow and easy. You'll need to do some extra checking on this guy and how he deals with personal relationships.

Encourage your man with loving words and touches. A warm smile and a word of encouragement can go a long, long way. Praise your man for his positive attributes. Express your appreciation for how thoughtful he is. Tell him you really respect how he attends to his familial obligations, that he can hold a job, and that he's dependable. Put the same amount of effort into praising him as you put into complaining about him.

We can't say this too many times:

Make sure that he knows that you like him. He should know by the loving attention you give him, but you must tell him often too!

Several of these types of dates should build a solid foundation on which to build a serious relationship. Eventually you will start to wonder if he might be "The One."

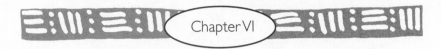
IF YOU REALLY THINK HE'S "THE ONE"

Word from the Brothahs

What makes a womban marriage material?

"I tell my sister, 'If a man likes you, you're gonna know.'"

"When it's true love, you know...this is right, this is the shit ...and you don't have to ask a lot of questions."

"If her concept of marriage is the same as mine and involves honesty, trust, dedication, things like this, then when she says to me, 'I want to get married,' I know what she's looking for ...what she's set out to do. She's set out to trust me and be there for me, like I would trust and be there for her."

"I think it was a little bit easier because I was giving out the signals. I'm a very communicative person. It didn't take long for somebody to realize where my head was at."

"Have I met 'The One'? I've met 'The One' two times already. They're gone now, and the thing of it is that if I had been ready, I'd be married [by now]. So if I meet the right person now, would I get married? Yes."

At this point you've been dating for a while and you are starting to wonder if he might be "The One," right? Well, seriously consider how you feel about him.

Do you love him?	**Y N**
Does he love you?	**Y N**
Do you trust him?	**Y N**
Does he feel the same way about you that you feel about him?	**Y N**

You should be able to answer "Yes" to all of these questions. If you can, then the timing of the proposal is partially in your control . . . but don't worry about that yet. We discuss how to actually get him to propose in "Poppin' the Question."

If you answered "No" to any of these questions, you should reconsider marriage with this guy. Answer the rest of the questions in this chapter and reevaluate your situation. If you have to kick him to the curb, then go back to the beginning of this book and start over. We don't want you to even *think* about marriage until you're *sure* you've got the right one, baby!

We realize that a lot of you who have been dating someone for years are opening the book to this page because you already think that you have "The One" on the hook. Well, we just want you to make sure that you *do* have "The *Right* One." First determine if your sweetheart is both ready to get married and appropriate for you, *then* decide how to manipulate the proposal. There could be several reasons why you two aren't engaged yet.

If you really think he's "The One," and you're not engaged yet,
   which one of you is holding up the proceedings?
————— HE IS   ————— I AM
Is it because you are not quite ready yourself?   **Y N**

Which category did you fit into when you took our twenty-five-question quiz?

A. You are ready.
B. You're almost ready.
C. You're *not* ready.
D. Don't even think about getting married . . . yet!

If you fit into category A or B, then you're one step ahead of the game and you just have to determine his readiness. If you fit into category C or D, then you need to identify and strengthen your weak areas.

Can You Determine If He's Ready?

If you're ready, maybe he's not. Can you determine if he's
   ready?   **Y N**

He's ready if . . . *he says he is*. If he doesn't know if he's ready, and you can't tell, then you need to evaluate him by answering the same questions about him that you answered about yourself in our twenty-five-question quiz. If you can't answer these questions about him, then you don't know him as well as you *think* you do. It's also a good idea to have him take the quiz himself, if he's ready, willing, and able. Then you can see how closely your assessments match.

Is He Ready?

This quiz gauges five aspects of his personality: spirituality, emotional stability, mental health, physical health, and cultural awareness. If he's been married before, use this quiz as well as the quiz in Chapter X. Reflect honestly in your answers—no wishful thinking. And if he takes the quiz, make sure he reflects honestly too.

Is He Ready Spiritually?

1. Is he centered? Does he feel whole and complete in his soul? **Y N**

2. Does he have a good solid relationship with his Creator/the Universe? **Y N**

3. Does he recognize positive energy that comes to him from close friends and relatives? **Y N**

4. Does he nourish his soul with natural beauty and positive people? **Y N**

5. Is he aware of the power of focused positive energy in his world? **Y N**

Is He Ready Mentally?

6. Is he aware of how his decision-making process works? **Y N**

7. Does he express himself clearly to others? **Y N**

8. Can he be bold, flexible, and decisive? **Y N**
9. Does he have any hobbies or interests outside his job? **Y N**
10. Is he willing to open himself to new experiences and new
    people in order to meet, greet, and keep a womban? **Y N**

Is He Ready Emotionally?

11. Has he ever been in love, that you know of? **Y N**
12. Does he love himself completely? **Y N**
13. Does he have ongoing loving, committed relationships
    with others? **Y N**
14. Can he tell the difference between true love and
    infatuation? **Y N**
15. Can he love unconditionally? **Y N**

Is He Ready Physically?

16. Has he had varied sexual experiences? **Y N**
17. Is he clear about his sexual orientation? **Y N**
18. Has he been in a long-term monogamous relationship? **Y N**
19. Is he where he wants to be in his life? **Y N**
20. Has he had an AIDS test? **Y N**

Is He Ready Culturally?

21. Does he know that our culture's herstory/history is not
    accurately represented in most educational systems? **Y N**
22. Is he aware of the varied social, scientific, and literary
    contributions made to our society by African Americans? **Y N**

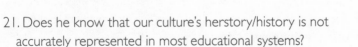

23. Is he aware of the hopelessness voiced in some of our young people's music? **Y N**

24. Does he actively seek ways to empower himself and his family and friends? **Y N**

25. A new Black Renaissance has emerged in our community at large. Has he read any Black scholarly work in the last year? **Y N**

Scoring and Working Out His Readiness

If he has "No" answers to

A. 0 questions: He is ready.

B. 1 to 5: He is almost ready.

C. 6 to 12: He's *not* ready.

D. 13 or more: He shouldn't even think about getting married...yet!

A. If he has "Yes" answers to most or all of the twenty-five questions, then he is seriously ready to get married.

B. If he has "No" answers to five or fewer questions, he still has some work to do on making himself a complete, happy, and mature man ready for commitment.

C. If he has "No" answers to six to twelve questions, you and he have a lot of other questions to answer, beginning with "Does he really want to get married? And if he does, *why* does he?" A careful and deep soul search will probably bring up issues that he has not dared look at before. Take it easy on him. Go slowly. There really is no rush. The only constraints he has are the ones he places on himself.

D. If he has "No" answers to thirteen or more questions, he's not close to knowing himself, never mind knowing whom or if he wants to marry.

You and he need to look closely and carefully at his motivations for seeking matrimony.

Note: If most of his no answers are in one category, he is probably neglecting one aspect of his personality. This doesn't mean that he's a hopeless case; it simply means that he has some work to do in one particular area of his life to get himself ready for that march down the aisle.

Many people are not able to answer yes to all of these questions by their Wedding Day, but through the caring, sharing, and growing that marriage entails, they will continue to develop the best in themselves.

Assessing His Appropriateness

Is it that he's not ready? Or is it that he's an inappropriate candidate for you? Or is it both?

_____

_____

_____

Appropriateness—whether he has the characteristics you are looking for in a man—is a totally different consideration from readiness. You have to get serious and determine if he is "The One" for you. This means that you must weigh all of his attributes against his faults and see how he measures up. This determination will help you decide if you want to spend the rest of your life with him.

There are no guarantees in life. I, Monique, was nervous as hell on my wedding day. Why? 'Cause even though Bobby was the greatest guy I'd ever met, how did I know he wasn't fronting? Even though he intended to live up to his wedding vows, maybe he wouldn't be able to . . . for reasons unknown to either of us. You can check him out thoroughly, but eventually you have to trust his actions *and* your ability to determine his true character. Answer the following questions to determine his appropriateness to the best of your ability.

1. Does he avoid "half-steppin' "?   **Y N**
2. Does he clearly communicate his feelings and thoughts to you?   **Y N**
3. Does he encourage you in all your endeavors?   **Y N**
4. Is he sincere in all his interactions with you?   **Y N**
5. Does he offer support when you are having serious problems?   **Y N**
6. Is he supportive and encouraging?   **Y N**
7. Does he share his resources with you as he's able, when necessary?   **Y N**
8. Does he voluntarily help out financially?   **Y N**
9. Does he occasionally splurge on you to show his appreciation?   **Y N**
10. Does he occasionally or spontaneously give you intimate, personal gifts?   **Y N**
11. Does he creatively suggest romantic rendezvous?   **Y N**
12. Is your sexual satisfaction a priority to him?   **Y N**

13. Does he try to reciprocate your nurturing and comforting? **Y N**

14. Does he uplift your spirits? **Y N**

15. Does he empathize when you need him to? **Y N**

16. Does he understand your needs? **Y N**

17. Does he voluntarily share in domestic chores? **Y N**

18. Does he cook for you? **Y N**

19. Does he match your emotional, physical, and spiritual commitment? **Y N**

20. Does he know how to give constructive criticism? **Y N**

21. Does he compliment you? **Y N**

22. Does he make you feel special? **Y N**

23. Is he considerate of your feelings? **Y N**

24. Does he (still) look at you with love and admiration? **Y N**

25. Does he have your "back"? **Y N**

Scoring and Working Out His Appropriateness

If you answered "No" to

A. 0 questions: He is appropriate.

B. 1 to 5: He is somewhat appropriate.

C. 6 to 12: He's *not* appropriate.

D. 13 or more: He'll never be appropriate.

A. If you answered "Yes" to all of the questions, then he really might be "The One." You should continue at the pace that seems to be working for the two of you. But first make sure to determine that although it may be taking a long time, he is in fact making sure and steady progress toward matrimony. He may offer a "promise ring" that signifies that within six to twelve months he will give you an actual engagement ring

 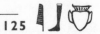

and that about a year from *that* date he will marry you. He probably needs this time to prepare himself for marriage. Only he can determine his own readiness and willingness to marry. Give him the space to decide when he is capable of making this lifelong commitment. It is essential that he feels that he has the freedom to decide without being pressured. Let him show you that during the course of your relationship, he has been making slow but steady steps toward the altar.

B. If you answered "No" to five or fewer questions, then he's just about ready to make the trek to the altar. Bide your time and keep talking and planning the way you have been. You'll soon find yourself having the final fitting of your wedding gown.

C. If you answered "No" to six to twelve questions, you'd better take a long hard look at what you want versus what you've got. You probably are a long way from having your daily needs met, never mind getting yourself to the altar!

D. If you answered "No" to half or more questions, forget about it! The guys, who ya'll have been seeing for three or more years without any indications of a proposed marriage ceremony, need to be "Cut Loose!"

Rate His Readiness *and* Appropriateness

The first letter in the left-hand column is his readiness category. The second letter is his appropriateness category. Combine the two letters to come up with his readiness and appropriateness rating. Check one answer:

AA ____ He is ready and appropriate.
AB ____ He is ready and somewhat appropriate.
AC ____ He is ready but *not* appropriate.

AD ____ He is ready but will never be appropriate.

BA ____ He is almost ready and is appropriate.

BB ____ He is almost ready and is somewhat appropriate.

BC ____ He is almost ready but is *not* appropriate.

BD ____ He is almost ready but will never be appropriate.

CA ____ He is not ready but he is appropriate.

CB ____ He is *not* ready but he is somewhat appropriate.

CC ____ He is not ready and not appropriate.

CD ____ He is *not* ready and will never be appropriate.

DA ____ He will never be ready or appropriate.

DB ____ He will never be ready but he is somewhat appropriate.

DC ____ He will never be ready and he is not appropriate.

DD ____ He will never be ready and will never be appropriate.

You should now have a pretty clear picture of your situation. In the following sections we give some advice for the most significant categories: AA, AB, BA, BB, and CA. If he falls into one of these categories, he is probably worth baggin'. If he falls anywhere else, *especially* CC or DD, *forget about him!* No exceptions.

AA He Is Ready and Appropriate

If he is ready and appropriate, and you're ready, are you not married because you haven't *discussed* marriage with him at all?

_____

Is he really "The One" but you don't want to change your life to accommodate the compromise and responsibility that a partnership demands?   **Y N**

So if he's ready and appropriate, then move on to the next chapter!

AB He Is Ready and Somewhat Appropriate

We realize that most of our girlfriends don't want to hear squat about how their man ain't been doing anything for them lately. But guess what? . . . If you are one of those girlfriends, we're here to tell you that you are missing out! By holding on to a guy that you *think* is "The One," you are in essence keeping the hands of fate from bringing your husband into your life. Make no mistake about it . . . how "yo' man" is . . . how he's been in the past few years, is exactly how he will handle the rest of your lives together. Don't be lulled into a false sense of security. Don't rationalize and think that if only you could get him to marry you, he'll change and everything will be different. You may not realize that it's not about the man anymore. It's more about your ego. You feel that in order to vindicate yourself for falling in love with him and spending so much time with him in the first place, you must prove (to yourself) that he can be "gotten" and that you can do the "gettin'." Look at it. Realize it. And let it go. You're wasting valuable time.

OK, he is ready but he's only somewhat appropriate. What are the qualities that make him unsuitable for you at this time?

_____

_____

_____

BA He Is Almost Ready and Is Appropriate

How many times have you heard that a girlfriend drop-kicked her man to the curb *after* she'd done her damnedest to get him just where she wanted him?!? Sometimes you may feel that even an on-again, off-again, familiar sex partner is better than nothing. How can we convince you of how vital it is to clear your psychic aura of the presence of this man's energy? He is keeping you from attracting your husband-to-be. Having the courage to get out of a long-standing and unfruitful relationship might be the single most important step you take in preparing yourself for marriage. Hello! . . . Are you listening? We may be talking to you.

If you still think he's really "The One," then why aren't you married yet?

_____

_____

_____

Are you waiting for him to pop the question in a manner that fulfills
your girlish romantic fantasies?   **Y N**

BB He Is Almost Ready and Is Somewhat Appropriate

If he's almost ready and is somewhat appropriate, you must determine how long you're willing to wait for him. If he's good enough for you and wants to get married in the near future, go for it—but only if you have a time frame that you're both aware of. Given this concrete time frame, as long as you stick to it, hang in there. Remember, he should show an obvious willingness to get married sometime soon.

Is he making small, but decisive "baby steps" toward
commitment and marriage to you?   **Y N**
Is he agreeing to specific ideas, dates, and budgets in planning
a wedding with you?   **Y N**
Is he suggesting that you look for a place together so you can
start pooling your resources to buy a house or pay for
the wedding?   **Y N**

CA He Is Not Ready but He Is Appropriate

If he's appropriate for you but not ready, let him go, 'cause remember he might be just fine for someone else. (If this makes you wince, remember that what goes around, comes around . . .)

Do you want to wait for him?   **Y N**
Why do you want to wait for him?

_____

_____

_____

Have you been involved with him for years as he dangles
marriage before you as a prize to be won at some future
date?   **Y N**
Has he followed through on the agreed-upon short-term
goals that pertain to your life together?   **Y N**

CC He Is *Not* Ready and *Not* Appropriate

If you *know* that he's not ready to get married or doesn't want to marry you, why are you wasting time?

_____

_____

_____

If he's *not* ready and he's *not* appropriate, bite the bullet and just dump him. Take some time to heal (the healing meditations in Chapter II will help a lot). Don't beat yourself up for having been in love with someone who was inappropriate. As you've matured, you've simply outgrown him. No shame, no blame. You're entitled to true happiness.

DD He Will Never Be Ready and Will Never Be Appropriate

Is he really *not* "The One," but you insist on forcing him into
   the mold of husband material?   **Y N**
Are you infatuated with him?   **Y N**

If "No," dump him!! If "Yes," get over it, 'cause you'll *never* marry a man you're infatuated with. Sorry, but thems the breaks. (See p. 25 for the difference between infatuation and love.)

Emotional Risk Investment

Do you simply want an "insertable" man? (That is, a man who
fits into your life just enough to satisfy most of your needs,
yet doesn't disrupt your routine or lifestyle.)   **Y N**

Or does he want an "insertable" womban in his life and you
haven't had the guts to tell him that you expect to be
more than that to him?   **Y N**

Do you want a man that you don't have to take care of
unless *you* want to.   **Y N**

Do you want what is popularly known as a "maintenance
man"? (That's a guy who comes around every now and
then to check your "plumbing" or who will give you a
good "lube job" when your private parts are a little "rusty.")   **Y N**

If you answered "Yes" to any of these questions, then you
need to reevaluate your own readiness and desire for marriage.
You may have a well-integrated personality and have even found
a man who is ready and appropriate, but you are not willing to
take the risks or make the compromises required to marry.

On pages 134–135 is a chart to help you determine your Emotional Risk Factor in your search for a mate. Your ability to make
a high-risk emotional investment is an indication of your readiness for the risks involved in committing to a man. What are you
willing to give up in order to win true love from a wonderful
husband?

It helps to understand the term "expected rate of emotional return." A high-risk emotional investment might be a situation like
dating a married man. A high emotional return would be that he

leaves his wife and family to marry you. But the likelihood of that happening is incredibly low, so your expected rate of return would be low. A more sensible, lower-risk emotional investment would be marrying "Mr. Right." The emotional return might be a happy marriage—a pretty likely occurrence. So your rate of emotional return will equal or surpass your initial emotional investment.

What kind of emotional risk do you think you're taking (or are you willing to take) in order to find happiness? Circle one:

ZERO   LOW   MODERATE   HIGH   EXTREME
RISK   RISK   RISK   RISK   RISK

Circle the type of emotional investment you wish to risk:

	ZERO RISK	LOW RISK	MODERATE RISK	HIGH RISK	EXTREME RISK
Staying single and alone	◎				
Platonic dating		◎			
Dating one person at a time with heavy pet-ting		◎			
Dating one person at a time with sex		◎			
Committing to the "in-sertable" man			◎		
Marrying Mr. Right			◎		
Staying single and adopting children			◎		
Dating more than one person with sex and using condoms				◎	

Where do you fall on the scale? Circle one:

ZERO RISK   LOW RISK   MODERATE RISK   HIGH RISK   EXTREME RISK

Are you willing to increase your emotional risk investment?   **Y N**

Are you willing to decrease your emotional risk investment?   **Y N**

Do you feel that your degree of investment is too great to start over?   **Y N**

Are you investing enough to get back the desired return?   **Y N**

	ZERO RISK	LOW RISK	MODERATE RISK	HIGH RISK	EXTREME RISK
Staying with Mr. Wrong hoping he'll turn into Mr. Right				◎	
Marrying or committing to lesbian Ms. Right				◎	
Living with Mr. Wrong or Mr. Right				◎	
Marrying Mr. Wrong				◎	
Having a child with but not marrying Mr. Wrong					◎
Having a child with but not marrying Mr. Right					◎
Dating more than one person with sex and not using condoms					◎
Dating married men					◎

His previous statements and actions, coupled with his and your responses to the questions in this chapter, should be enough to let you know whether or not to continue with the relationship. If not, just go back a few chapters and start looking for another prospect! If so, then you should be well on your way to married bliss! We'd say that you're ready for a more intimate rendezvous!

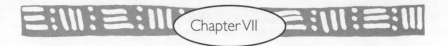

Chapter VII

LeT's TAlk AbOuT sEx!

Word from the Brothahs

How early is too soon for a prospective wife to go to bed with you?

"Never too soon."

"Don't sleep with a man until after you're married."

"I might be one of those corny guys or something, but my feeling is, I don't expect any of that the first couple of dates."

Do you practice safer sex?

"Sometimes."

"All the time.

"No."

"Everybody should have an AIDS test before they get together."

"Oh, yes. I believe in taking an AIDS test. It's very important ...and I want to see her ID too."

Why don't you call after sex?

"A womban shouldn't sleep with a man and then just sit around and wait for the phone to ring. If she feels like calling, she should call. The wait for that phone call is equally shared."

"I might talk to her on the phone ten times before we even touch each other, but it's a level of conversation that you have…each time it gets deeper and deeper, and you're communicating. The telephone is a serious instrument."

"If the womban is confident, and the womban's happening, I'm gonna be there the next morning so I don't have to call her."

"I've gone out with womben and stuck with womben because the sex was good [knowing that they weren't about too much] but it was good…and they did things that *good* girls didn't do."

How do you feel about oral sex?

"You can't ask an old person that. Old people don't—we don't answer those questions."

"A lot of womben want it but they don't know how to ask for it."

"Some womben are afraid to do it. They think you're gonna ask them 'Where you learn how to do that?'"

"If she's willing to fulfill my desires, then I'm willing to fulfill hers. Bottom line."

HOT STUFF

Sex is the window through which two lovers allow their souls the chance to meet and dance among the stars. This rapturous event can be the culmination of many hours of personal interchange, or it can be the result of a moment's impetuous embrace. Be prepared to witness the power of this passion. It has the ability to change your life—if it is experienced wholeheartedly. It can uplift you, but only if you don't have too many expectations. The secret is to just enjoy it. Great sex is not just screwing. It is the intimate exchange of natural love which promotes physical bonding. It's the intermingling of hot, sweaty, excited bodies. A flow of intimate feelings evolves out of an erotic awareness.

Have you ever had really great sex?   **Y N**

Describe your most sensuous experience.

_____

_____

_____

Erotica is the stuff that turns you on. It can be the ultimate aphrodisiac, used to enhance your sexual encounters. Things that you may find erotic are, for example, taking a sensual bath with bubbles, essential oils, herbs, or flower petals in a tub surrounded by lit candles; being massaged or oiled by your lover; having your feet caressed and kissed; promising your next move via suggestive whispers . . .

Come

Come…

Flow with me…like water.

Whispers in my ear…

Swim with me…

Let me pound like waves onto your shore,

While waves of passion swell.

Cresting…

Crashing onto the beach…

Foaming…

Roiling into the sand…

Into crevices of corals and rocks.

Come…

Flow with me…like water.

Swim with me in your ocean,

Carry me upon your waves

To places I've never been.

Come…flow with me…

Like water.

Erotica is things that you can see and hear and taste. Music colors the mood. Don't restrict yourself to soft romantic tunes. Keep in mind the throbbing beat of the dance floor.

What are your favorite par-tay songs?

_____

_____

_____

Our inheritance of rhythms that resonate deep within our souls are gifts from our ancestors that transcend time. Don't squander this gift by tapping into it only in public. Remember Tina Turner's "Private Dancer"? Give a command performance for your lover one night. If you have qualms about "appearing" nude for him, just think of these profound words: "When you're the only naked womban in the room, you've got center stage . . . *and baby you're a star!*" So let him, as Prince says, "be the *Big Dipper!*"

What are your apprehensions about performing or doing something wild for your mate?

_____

_____

_____

Do you think that he might not be receptive to your
overtures? **Y N**

Is his idea of erotic stimulation cuddling up and watching
car racing together? **Y N**

Remember: Every couple has their own ideas about what's sexy and what turns them on.

Ask him about his fantasies. There might be one that you could fulfill that will start you on your way to a little more sensuality in your life. As for your own fantasies, you don't need validation for what turns you on. It's personal. So let your imagination run wild.

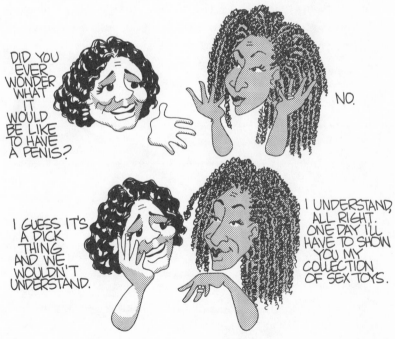

But if you want to start with something tamer, maybe you need a less direct approach—like writing a "foreplay letter."

A "foreplay letter" is a steamy love letter intended to turn him on. All you have to do is recount one of the great times you've had in bed with him, including all the details that you have to leave out when you're "givin' the girls the 411" on him. Maybe in one of your subsequent letters you can describe one of your fantasies to him. Don't have any fantasies on tap? Then make one up. It's a fantasy, remember?

Perhaps you can coax him to write a foreplay letter to you. Have him put one of his fantasies on paper, write down something he'd like to try that he doesn't have the nerve to ask you for. Or have him read one of *your* letters to you. This will work well if you can't get him to write one to you. At least you get to hear his voice saying all those sexy things!

Detail a fantasy or write a foreplay letter for him to read to you.

_____

_____

_____

_____

_____

Read to each other, in and out of bed, but especially in bed. There are a few Black erotic books available that would be a great addition to any library (see our recommended reading list). Draw a nice bubble bath. Get in. Alone or together. Take turns reading short erotic poems to each other. Or on a Sunday morning in bed, instead of reading the *Sunday News,* try reading some poetry, something that expresses your feelings for each other, something that caught your eye and made you think of the other. It doesn't matter whether the poems are reflective of what *you* feel or what you think *he* might feel. Don't worry if you think you don't *get* poetry. If it sounds good . . . feels good . . . then . . . do it!

Here's one to try: Ask him if he'd make breakfast for you one Sunday mornin'. After he's gotten up and started going into the kitchen, follow him in your sexiest negligee while saying in your most sultry voice . . . "hey baby . . ."

What's Cookin'?

When I'm near you, my body heats up

like Mama's skillet

when it's licked by those cool blue flames.

First the center starts to glow,

radiating heat into an ever-widening circle.

As the color of that hot black thing changes,

An unmistakable scent arises. Indescribable.

Promising tastes and satisfaction for the most discerning tongue.

Impatiently watching

water droplets dance across its hot surface,

Sizzling & popping

Testing the vessel for readiness.

You just might end up being the appetizer or the dessert. Another great turn-on using literature, if you or your guy speaks or reads another language fluently, is to read in that language. Try a love poem!

Now that we have tantalized your senses with how it can be, let's address the issues of when you should indulge in such stimulating pleasures. To do it, or not to do it? That is the question. Making the decision to have sex with someone is a very personal and intimate decision. No one can tell you when the "right" time is. The so-called sexual revolution has left us with no real rules of conduct. These days almost anything goes! Whether you sleep with him on the first date or wait until the Wedding Night... you're *still* considered a lady. Only you and your partner know what's appropriate.

We suggest doing the *wild thang* sooner rather than later. Why so soon? So that you know if you're sexually compatible regarding preferences of frequency, chemistry, duration, time, location, and all of the other important details that go into making sex happenin' for you.

Do you really want to spend the rest of your life with
someone who's lousy in bed?!?   **Y N**

Or maybe he's just not used to doing the things to you that you like done. Perhaps he doesn't take direction well. He just might be a younger man with limited sexual experience. Whatever, you must be able to talk frankly with each other about your sex life.

We realize that sex can improve as people grow together and feel more comfortable with each other. But by starting early you find out *before* you fall in love... or at least early enough so that you don't have to make it obvious that his sexual prowess (or lack thereof) is the only reason you're drop-kicking him to the curb.

Special note: When doing the *wild thang*, make sure that he calls you by *your* name! Baby, Sugah, Mama, Sweet Thang, and other endearments are cute and sexy, but he could be using those names on some other

"Honey"! One way to encourage him to address only you is to use his name at the moment of no return.

Safer Sex

Of course you're practicing safer sex! If a guy tells you he doesn't use condoms, then you know he's not "The One." If he's not using condoms with you, then he probably didn't use them with his previous partners. Risky business. If he cares about himself, he should be using them. If he cares about you, he will.

After you've found out whether you're sexually compatible you can go have an AIDS test together. People have been known to lie about their HIV status or test results. You'll be assured that you're not getting into something you may not be able to handle. (Of course, this doesn't mean that you stop performing safer sex, it just means that you'll both have more peace of mind.)

How do you bring up the topic of safer sex and the AIDS test with someone you hardly know? You just do! Ask him *"Are you dating anyone else?" "How intimate are you?" "Have you been sexually active recently?" "With how many people?" "What kind of sexual acts did you perform with them?" "Did you use latex?"*

Sometimes this is a very good place to begin your sexual fantasy foreplay. Imagining you're a news reporter or night nurse can get your head into a different space. If you're not really yourself asking these questions, sometimes they're easier to deal with. But, remember, if you can't communicate verbally, how can you communicate sexually?

Hint: This may be one of those times that you role-play with one of your girlfriends. You can take turns practicing asking each other these kinds of questions.

You also want to be able to talk openly and honestly with the man who is potentially going to be your best friend. The best times to do this are when you're en route from one place to another. Say, after dinner, you take a little walk. This would be a good time to bring up the topic. Or on your way to or from that movie. Don't wait until you've started necking and the temperatures are rising. By then it's usually too late.

Have you both been tested for the HIV virus?   **Y N**
Seen each other's results?   **Y N**

If not, then your next date should be at the clinic! So what if you've been celibate for the last two years? And *he* swears that he hasn't been with anyone since his ex-wife? You should make sure you know where you stand. If the issue is trust, then this can be proof that you do trust each other.

Latex can be fun! Just remember to have plenty of lubrication jelly on hand (some of you older Sistahs may be pleasantly surprised at how a little lube can facilitate activities!). Make sure that you use a water-based lube and not a petroleum-based one (such as Vaseline, baby/mineral/vegetable oil), because non-water-based lubes can break down the latex.

Using latex gloves for hand jobs—his and hers—can introduce an element of kinkiness to the sexual act. Questions like *"Do you want to play doctor tonight? You be the patient"* or *"Dr. Love, I need an examination. Do you think you can help me?"* are fun and playful.

Have you ever considered using role-playing as a part of
   your sexual life?   **Y N**

If you want him to go down on you, but he's acting or feeling
a little leery (and it's not that Black male chauvinist junk), then
just pull out the Saran Wrap. Yes, Saran Wrap (or whatever brand
of plastic wrap you use). It has to be the *nonmicrowavable* type
(nonporous), but it works fine as a handy dental dam. Plus, you
don't have to go crazy trying to find the damn dams at the drug-
store or local slinky sex shop! Just tear off a healthy piece of
wrap, one that's long enough to be anchored by your butt, and
hold the top end. Then let your partner go to work!

In the case of giving head to him, you simply need a supply of
nonlubricated condoms. Either ask your druggist, or go to one
of those big drugstores where they have walls of condoms. Then
go to town, Sis! *Give head!* All men would kill for it at one time
or another. One good thing about giving head with a condom is
that you can be a little more creative with your teeth. We defy
any man to say that he can't feel *that!* (Use a flavored condom—
they're fun!) If you're not good at it at first, it doesn't matter. Men
don't care as long as you try! Eventually you'll get used to it and
get better at it. Black men think, "If you *really* care about me
you'll do it." You may even come to like it, especially when you
see how ecstatic it makes him! You don't have to deep throat
him, just put it in your mouth and suck on it like a popsicle. Lick
it, slurp it . . . enjoy it! When in doubt . . . *ask!!* "Am I doing it
right?" or "How do you like it?" Trust me, he'll let you know.
He'll be glad you asked. He may even be surprised that you care
enough to ask. And who knows, one good turn deserves another
. . . what goes around, *comes* around!

Special note: If you're good at giving head, you might want to save it for that special someone or for a special time. If you don't know whether you're good at it or not, you probably need practice. If you need more instructions about this or any other sexual activities, check out *The Joy of Sex* and its sequels or any other reputable (or disreputable) books. Large bookstores usually have walls of books on sexuality. The next time you're bored, or want an exciting date, slide on down to the bookstore and check out some new material. (Erotic videos also work well for getting ideas.)

Sex books can help you become more uninhibited by giving you fresh ideas. Having new ideas and positions will also help you become more assertive in bed. Some Black men love to be made love to (try it in front of mirrors), to have the womban approach them and take control in bed. Astonishing, but true, most men want a whore in the bedroom and a lady everywhere else.

Note: Don't worry about following all the rules in the sex manuals or our sexual advice. It doesn't matter whether you're having a mental orgasm, a physical orgasm, a clitoral orgasm, or a vaginal orgasm; as long as you're having fun, honey, don't worry about it! Sex is mental. Intimacy and foreplay are equally important to the act of love. Orgasm can be like getting the brass ring on the merry-go-round of sexual intercourse. But don't forget to enjoy the ride before concentrating on the extra prize.

Talking during sex turns Black men on. They love to hear your fantasies. Don't be afraid to tell him what you want, need, like, or might be curious about. If you usually make a lot of noise during sex, try remaining silent or holding in your noises. If you're usually silent, let out a couple of bloodcurdling screams. Ditto for your level of participation: If you usually lie there not moving much, make a concerted effort to try a new position, shake your derriere. If you're always all over the place, take it slow and easy, and for once just lie back and enjoy it. Remember: "A change is better than a rest."

Hint: No matter what size his is, always tell him *"Wow, what a big, beautiful penis you have!"* Most men are normally endowed, but the myth of the "Big Black Buck" makes them wonder if they measure up to the competition. You'll be soothing his anxieties by assuring him that he's just right for you.

Does he please you? How?

_____

_____

_____

_____

Tell him! Tell him what you like to do to him. Then ask him to return the favor. Reminisce over past episodes with him (even if you've only done *it* together a couple of times). Laugh about any disasters or bumpy places. (Don't forget that humor goes a long way in keeping a relationship going over the rough spots.)

Finally, make sure that you and he are alone—mentally—during sex. Don't bring your parents, former lovers, past sexual experiences, his ex-wife, or your critical inner voice to bed with you. They can be most inhibiting to your sex life.

It's OK to Go Straight

At some time or another we have all put ourselves into categories of sexual identity. Climbing into a box or assigning yourself a label that defines who you are feels safe and comfortable. In fact, it is a powerful and liberating thing to name yourself. But what happens if sometime you decide to climb into a different box or change your label? Or maybe add more labels? What if you've settled in a box that your family and friends can't relate to? That you yourself don't understand?

Don't let honest fear and self-doubt hold you back from contentment. The key is to determine what your needs are and how best to fulfill them. Sometimes this has to be determined by trial and error. It shouldn't be scandalous to honestly explore your sexuality. In her book *Vice Versa,* Marjorie Garber explains how the exciting influence of bisexuality has infiltrated our society in a big way! She documents how the extensive use of bisexual images to sell all sorts of products directly influences our psyches. If you aren't conscious of these influences, sharpen your awareness by recognizing the broad use of androgynous models in the media. Note the mixed messages society is sending.

In what way is your previous life choice relevant to your present situation?

_____

_____

Have you ever labeled yourself a lesbian or bisexual? **Y N**

If not, how do you label yourself?

_____

_____

Does this label affect your perception of your new
  relationship with a man? **Y N**

If so, how?

_____

_____

What fears do you have about changing your sexual identity?

_____

_____

The time is always ripe to unlock hidden desires. You cannot
allow outside influences to determine your life choices. Discover
how to transform yourself. This requires earnest dedication to
your principles and clarity of thought. If you think that you
would be happy married to a man, go for it. You have an obliga-
tion to yourself to find out.

How do you plan to garner emotional support for your transformation?

_____

_____

_____

_____

_____

_____

_____

Do what *you've* gotta do. You can find support for whatever your life choices are. Many anthologies, magazines, newsletters, groups, and organizations exist that will offer you information about whatever changes you're going through. You are not alone. Of course, you won't find any help if you don't look for it! You have to work a *little* harder to find what you're looking for, and you might not have everything you want all at the same time, but like the old Stones' song, "You can't always get what you want . . . but you can try sometimes . . . to get what you need."

The Waiting Game

Waiting for "that call" after the hottest sex you've ever had has got to be the most stressful experience that a single womban faces in our oh-so-modern times. We say, *if he doesn't call in the next day or so . . . forget about him!* Don't drive yourself crazy imagining a million scenarios of why he can't get to the phone. Our research has shown that if he really cared about you (and not just the sex), he would call right away. No ifs, ands, or buts about it! Move on to the next victim/candidate. Two weeks later when the chucklehead finally does call (because he cares about the great sex and not you), tell him in no uncertain terms that you're busy, baby, and to get over it—'cause you did!

On the other hand, praise your man for his positive attributes, including his sexual prowess, as often and sincerely as you are able. "Sexual healin'" goes a long way. Let's face it, sex is the only thing we have left that hasn't been made Eurocentric. "They" have always looked to us for the "mo better" way to "knock the boots" and "they" probably always will. So give credit where credit is due.

So if you think that you've checked him out thoroughly, both in and out of bed, then it's time to talk about *poppin' the question!*

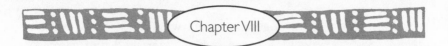

Chapter VIII

POPPIN' THE QUESTION

Word from the Brothahs

Do you think you must have a ring in hand to propose?

"No."

"I think so."

"It's exciting, but not necessary."

"I don't think it's necessary."

"No."

"No. I don't feel that way, but her father felt that way."

Would it matter if she asked you to marry her?

"No."

"No. Next question."

"No."

"If she asked me to marry her I would think she really cared and I would be impressed. I might go for it."

"If she says, 'Hey, I want to get married,' I think that's cool."

"I think more womben ask men to marry than men ask womben. That's my opinion."

You must first acknowledge to yourself what kind of guy you are dealing with. Would his ego be hurt if you asked him to marry you? If not, *ask him to marry you!* It's that simple. Just because *you* actually "popped the question" doesn't mean that you forbid him from planning some surprising, romantic way of showing you that he is madly in love with you. You've only taken some of the pressure off what can be a stressful decision for a man trying to say, "I'd like to spend the rest of my life with you." Halle Berry asked her husband, Atlanta Braves star Dave Justice, to marry her.

Many Black men feel they must perform some magic feat of romance. It doesn't have to be like that. All we really want is a special moment carved out of time to remember when the man of our dreams decided to announce to the world that he thinks we're special enough to love forever. Right?

Well, most men don't see it that way. They believe they must live up to the reputations of all the most romantic suitors history has ever produced. They have this insane notion that they have to be the next sexy, romantic superhero, slayer of dragons, and man about town, all rolled into one, right at the very moment they make this pledge of committed love. As if this is the only time in their entire lives that this behavior is possible! And, let's face it, they probably get these mixed signals from us. You have to convince them that they really don't have to go there.

How? By saying, "Hey, you know I don't expect any crazy surprise proposal or anything, honey. If you ever decide that you can't live without me, just let me know straight up. We're in this together. I think my world would never be the same without you. What about you?"

We've discovered from our research that half the time, that's the way it's done. Proposals are not always straightforward. He may not get down on his knee with ring and roses in hand. It's more likely that while you're having conversations about marriage, you'll have to listen carefully for cues. Instead of saying, "Yes," you might be saying, "Did you just say what I think you said?" You just might be getting a proposal.

Once the two of you agree that you're both ready *and* appropriate for each other and marriage, you might want to try the more traditional "wait and see when *he* pops the question" approach. Getting him to ask you to marry him takes a great deal of confidence and patience. You must make your serious intentions known to him, beyond a shadow of a doubt . . . and then you just have to wait.

Have you had "The Conversation" about the "M" word a
couple of times?   **Y N**

If not, then do so. How will you know he's willing to enter into an "exclusive engagement" with you if you don't discuss it? Don't hold in your true feelings. He may be waiting for a sign from you.

Are you afraid that you'll scare him off?   **Y N**

Don't be. If he runs, good riddance! However, timing has a lot to do with pulling this off successfully. Generally speaking, don't ask him to marry you on the first date! But if you think the climate is appropriate, it's perfectly OK to bring up marriage or the fact that you're looking for a husband on the first date. It's up to you and your particular Black man.

Make No Bones About Your Quest

On our first date I, Monique, told the man I would later marry that I was in search of a husband. I said that he was a nice guy and all that, but no way would I even consider him as marriage material because he was way too young. We could keep dating . . . but even if he wanted to marry me, I wouldn't take him seriously! He just looked at me deadpan for a minute and then replied, "Don't underestimate me." "Good answer," I thought, and five years, two kids, and one book later I'm still quite rapturously married to him. The point, as we've tried to make clear throughout this book, is that *it's not what you say but how you feel when you're saying it*. By now you should have the confidence to realize that if it doesn't work out with this particular guy, you are such a desirable package that you will find the right man.

It's safe to say that after a year or two, the time is right. If he's commitment phobic, better to know now than waste any more time with him. Just go back to the beginning of the book and start beating the bushes for another bird (candidate)!

After you've had "the Conversation," you have to sit back. Give *him* a window of opportunity and trust that he'll "do the right thing." This is the opening curtain of the biggest, most important (and maybe the only) full-scale production of your life to date. We will give you some scenarios and some direction, but like any good improvisation, you have to come up with the script that's appropriate to the situation. Use your common sense and best judgment. If you truly feel that you are ready to share your life with this man, don't ignore your intuition and instinct about communicating this to him. Trust yourself as much as you trust him. That makes for a great beginning, no matter how you look at it.

Setting the Scene

There are several ways to get a guy to "pop the question," all of which start out the same way . . . by *letting him know* how serious you are about being married. His sincere interest in getting married has to be evident before you begin. You've spent a good amount of time together, so you have an idea of how he thinks and feels. *How* you make him aware of your intentions advances his likeliness to propose.

Make It Happen

If he wants to marry you, he'll ask. The trick is letting him know that you're ready without sounding like you're giving him an ultimatum. You have to give him the space to feel that it's (at least partially) his idea in the first place. This implies successfully manipulating his feelings so he wants to make the plunge into wedded bliss. Let's get one thing clear right now: There is nothing wrong with manipulation. We all manipulate people, feelings, and things *every day* to reach our personal goals. This is not bad! For some reason society has decided that it's bitchy to be able to "manipulate" effectively. Perhaps because womben are so fierce at it? Men see manipulation as a win-or-lose situation. They have been taught to believe that if they are manipulated to any end (knowingly or unknowingly) they lose. They win only if they resist manipulation, even if the ultimate outcome is beneficial to them. This is the crux of the proposal issue. Men hate being manipulated, period. Especially when it comes to marriage. So the key is to make him *think* it's his idea to get married in the first place.

You have by this time *opened the circuit* in his brain that allows him to consider marriage as a place he wants to be. He's amazed (maybe appalled) that he hasn't run. He's surprised that it doesn't sound like a bad idea to be married . . . to you. Since you are the one who's enabled him to entertain the idea, he naturally *connects* the concept with you! He may balk, because that's what men are *supposed* to do, but he's finding that it's really *not* such a bad idea.

Now that you know this secret about Black men, you must devise a clever way to get your partner to realize that being manipulated by you on this and any other issue is and will always be the best thing that could ever happen to his life. In our estimation, agreeing to marry implies an eager desire on his part to be manipulated and on your part to manipulate him, and vice versa, openly and honestly.

Speaking hypothetically is another effective way to convince him of just how earnest you are. For example, saying things like "If we were married, my mother wouldn't get so upset every time she comes to visit" or "If I had gotten pregnant when I was single I think I would have kept the baby, but now that my feelings for you have grown so deep, if I got pregnant now, I don't know what I'd do. I wouldn't want you to think that I'm trying to keep you by getting pregnant. But being single *and* in love with you would make it a much harder decision to make." There must be an element of seriousness in the hypothetical remarks you make during your conversations about marriage. Your calculated comments must be designed to convince him how badly you wish to be married to him, without pressuring him. Be careful, ladies, this requires a delicate balancing act, but we are sure that you can pull it off. We can't tell you exactly what to say because each relationship is unique and these important comments must be tailor-made to fit your particular man, relationship, and situation. But we *can* point you in the right direction.

What is the tailor-made comment or question you can pose to your man that will convince him of just how serious you are about marrying him?

_____

_____

Pride Goeth Before a Fall

Your pride can stand in the way of your successful endeavor. Don't let a certain mindset or pattern of behavior stop you from getting what you want. Don't be a stubborn fool about unimportant things. Compromise. You have to. That's one of the major challenges of marriage anyway.

As we've already advised, however, one way to avoid all the hassle and uncertainty is to do the poppin' yourself! This is the simplest, most direct way to get what you want.

Cassandra Proposed to Her Husband

And it worked! I asked my husband to marry me. We were sitting around talking about our individual futures. He was telling me his goals: He wanted to live in the States after he finished his studies, and he would then tour the world as a "top musician." I shared my dreams with him while we continued to date, hanging out, sharing good times.

As he was a foreigner, I was naturally concerned about his ability to stay in the country, both legally and financially. He, at this point, shared with me that his government was paying his complete tuition for him to earn his degree in the States—all expenses paid for the duration. So I asked him if he wanted to get married to stay in the country for a little while after he graduated.

He turned me down cold. He told me that although he loved his experiences here, he had decided to marry for love. I said that I respected that and understood, since I had already married for love once and knew what beautiful experiences it contained. So we continued to date and share good times.

One night, similar to many nights at home, "the Conversation" arose again. He mentioned the word *Love*. I proposed to him, as I had once before. It wasn't hard to ask again. This time he accepted. We planned the wedding, an elopement, for after Christmas and Kwanzaa celebrations. I told only my two best friends. I didn't tell my mom or sisters, not even my twelve-year-old son or Monique. I chose Sadie Hawkins Day, February 29, 1988.

Still thinking and feeling that I was such a "radical" for eloping, I found myself a few weeks later, on my wedding night,

How to Marry a Black Man

looking into that Brothah's eyes and being deeply and blissfully "in love." Eight years and a daughter later, we're still hangin'.

So, you see, it *is* possible to pop the question yourself. On the other hand, what if you have the guy, you have the will and the inclination, but you don't have the guts, and you just *have* to know if he'll marry you? What's a womban to do!?! You can always talk to his best friend to gauge how he's feeling about matrimony, or, if you're close to any of his family members, you might try talking to them. But unless he himself knows for sure what he needs, his intentions could remain a mystery indefinitely. If you can't ask him and he won't tell, you may just have to wait patiently.

Engagement Rings

It's also wise to put his fears to rest about having to provide an expensive engagement ring—unless you simply refuse to get married without one! The customary equation for determining the price of the engagement ring is one to two months of the groom's salary. There are many other affordable options, including the traditional diamond/gold engagement ring. We've found that the cost for diamond rings runs the gamut, from a preowned pawnshop gem to a top-of-the-line rock—anywhere from $200 to $10,000. Therefore, we will explain the determining factors, which we outline as the *five C's*. The fifth *C*—the cost—depends on the other four.

Cut: Shapes can be marquis, heart, teardrop, princess, radiant, trillion, and round. They're all desirable cuts; the value is in your personal taste.

Color: The color of a diamond is white. The more colorless-white it is, the more valuable it is. A blue-white classification in diamonds does not exist.

Clarity: An absence of imperfections or particles increases the value.

Carat: The heavier the stone, the higher the value. In the price range of $200 to $10,000, the weight varies from one-quarter point to one point.

Diamond engagement rings are more affordable than most people think. Depending on his budget, he can purchase a decent ring starting at about two thousand dollars. Be wary of going to an unfamiliar jeweler to buy a good diamond ring. Try to find someone you know you can trust. Depend on word of mouth to locate a reputable jeweler. *Engagement Rings: the Definitive Buying Guide for People in Love* by Antoinette Matlins will help you out tremendously. Also call Tiffany & Co. at 1-800-526-0649 for a complimentary copy of *How to Buy a Diamond.*

You don't have to have a diamond ring. One girlfriend had the opportunity to create her own wedding band and engagement ring out of yellow gold and a beautiful freshwater pearl. Her husband had a friend who was a jeweler. So they all sat down and designed a ring together. She now has a unique set of rings. Any gemstone set in gold or silver would make an affordable, but exquisite engagement ring.

If you and your man are seriously strapped for cash or don't really care about having or wearing a traditional ring, you may want to consider using his college ring; or maybe there is a family heirloom that can be passed down. There are many ways to get a ring. Just don't let the issue of a ring keep you from getting hitched. We've found that many Black couples get engaged (and married) without an engagement ring. A ring can be presented eventually, as an anniversary or birthday gift, but it's not essential for a romantic pledge of love and commitment.

Baby Matters

An age-old method for baggin' a Brothah, iffy at best, is the old "I'm pregnant" routine. This one often backfires, especially if you intentionally get pregnant just to "trap" him. But if you are willing to risk *your* life, the life of your child, the life of your intended, *and* your good relationship with him, go ahead. Be prepared to hear later, "I only married you because you were pregnant."

Can you live with that for the rest of your life?   **Y N**

If your pregnancy was sincerely an accident, and you believe him to be a potentially great father and husband, *tell him that you're pregnant.* You can only hope he will do the right thing by asking for your hand in marriage. The major problem with this scenario is that he may be ready to be a husband but not a father, or ready to be a father but not a husband. Only he can decide if he wants to take on the added responsibility *all at once.* Give him time to adjust to the idea. Don't pressure him into giving you an answer right away. Definitely tell him first, before you tell your families. He will appreciate the lead time to get his act together. Timing is everything. Then just chill and wait and see how he responds.

If he tells you right up front that he doesn't want to have anything to do with you or the child, forget about him and don't look back. It may be difficult, but you *will* find a way for you and your child. Necessity is the ultimate mother of invention. She will help you figure things out. Be mature and take responsibility for your actions and decisions. In this day and age, you don't really need him. Of course he would be a great asset for you as well as for your child. But if he is unwilling to participate on *any* level in the life of his child, "See ya!"

Describe what you will gain, besides money, by dragging him to paternity court?

_____

_____

If you can get financial support from him, do so. But realize that it will be a never-ending, uphill emotional battle that will constantly tempt you into believing that maybe one day he'll want to "claim" his child. We advise detaching emotionally as soon as humanly possible. Get the cash and dash.

He may, however, surprise you and offer to create a stable union in which to birth and raise your child. This is the right thing for him to do. Even if he responds favorably to your predicament, you must still give him time and space to practice juggling these new developments. Don't crowd him just because he's agreed to marry you. Be prepared for him to vacillate. Even the greatest guy is gonna waver under this kind of pressure. It certainly separates the boys from the men, regardless of age. The baby has to be viewed as an unexpected wedding present, not the culmination of the relationship. You must keep a clear understanding that the marriage is based on mutual love, understanding each other's strengths and weaknesses, and a mutual intent to marry, even if there were no *bambino*.

Living Together

Some people think that living together is a surefire method of leading him to the altar. We disagree. Most of the time it is as fu-

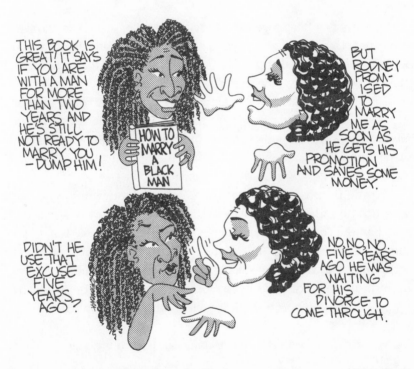

tile as the pregnancy route. If you don't agree to some "contractual terms" in place of a marriage certificate, then you simply have no bargaining power. Often womben are so excited about having a man committing to them on any level that they don't consider all that they are forgoing.

Living together can and does work *if* right from the beginning you set certain ground rules:

1. He is fully aware that you want to get married, to him, one day in the not-so-distant future.
2. He too wants to get married, to you, one day in the not-so-distant future.
3. He knows that living together is strictly a *temporary* situation and that you expect to be married by a certain date. Yes, this is an ultimatum! You set the time frame and stick to it. Make sure he knows that you're prepared to *get up and go* if he doesn't get his act together.
4. Maintain some thread of independence, such as a room at your mother's or at a girlfriend's even if you never really go there. This option, while largely psychological, makes all the difference in the world and is worth the extra bucks.

After he proposes and sets a date or gives you a ring, you can give up the independent place and start socking away some extra change. This is not technically "living" with him—but that's the point. He's aware that there's still a chance you could get away until and unless he makes you feel secure enough to move in and lose most of your negotiating power. Otherwise it doesn't usually end up like you think it will—with a wedding date.

Do you think that living with him is luring him toward the altar?   **Y N**

Remember what the old folks say: "Why buy the cow when you can get the milk for free?" By living together, you are both allowing yourselves to find out the worst things about each other without a *no back-out clause*—one of the things a marriage certificate is good for. Studies from three countries including the U.S. have shown that couples who cohabit prior to marriage have a higher divorce rate than those who don't.

Living together is a direct result of our desire for instant gratification borne out of the Me generation. By living together you think that you're satisfying needs for commitment and companionship. You're not. You're simply delaying maturity, real commitment, a positive self-image/self-esteem, and other opportunities for self-knowledge that are the essential building blocks of marriage.

Let's get down to the real nitty-gritty. We're not saying *never* live with a guy. Just don't live with a guy that you think you might want to marry—unless, of course, you've already got your ring and are saving *together* for a house or wedding expenses. Living in is a good way to learn about yourself: how to interact, share, and compromise. But it's not a good way to get married.

However, if you find yourself in that situation at present, what do you do? You're gonna have to make a few hard decisions, like whether you have anything to lose by delivering an ultimatum—"We get married within the next —— months, or I'm outta here!" Be willing to stand by such a declaration of your needs because a threat is useless if you're unwilling to carry it out!

Why are you staying in this tenuous situation when what you really want is a marital commitment?

_____

_____

_____

Is the reason primarily financial?   **Y N**
   Or is it the "comfort zone"?
Are you afraid of pushing too hard and losing him?   **Y N**
What are you giving up in the bargain?   **Y N**
Are you comfortable waiting an indefinite number of months
   or years more?   **Y N**
How old are you? Is your biological clock ticking?   **Y N**

List the pros and cons of staying in the living-in situation:

Pros:

_____

_____

Cons:

_____

_____

How do they balance out?

_____

_____

Are you really getting what you need and deserve by staying
in this situation? **Y N**

We don't usually recommend handing out ultimatums, but this
is one situation where it's appropriate. You're just stalling by
staying in an open-ended relationship. He's probably telling you
that he'll marry you . . . someday. But, Honey, time's a'wastin'!!!
Before you issue your ultimatum, you'd better have a new living
space mapped out. Who knows, when you move out, maybe another one of those old folks' sayings will hold true as well: "You
never miss the water till the well runs dry." He *may* realize what
he's lost . . . and propose.

If you're letting financial constraints determine your emotional
disposition, then you need to check out your true needs and desires. There are other types of living situations that are economi-
cal but that leave you free to pursue your true emotional goals.
Roommates and house sharing help keep expenses down. Many
elderly or retired folks are willing to rent a room to a single
womban for a nominal fee. House sitting and caretaking newsletters carry information about obtaining these kinds of situations,
which are virtually cost-free.

It's not always easy, but sometimes living with parents or sib-
lings can be a way to save for your own property. There are

many houses on the market today, especially in older, less fashionable neighborhoods, that come with a very low mortgage.

You know who he is and when he'll be there. There's a warm bod to snuggle up to. Regular safer sex is on the menu. And, hopefully, you only have to pay half of the bills!?!

But how comfortable are you really, not being married?

_____

_____

If he won't take that next, logical step to matrimony, how comfortable can it be for you? If he's not the one, but you're living together, you don't have the space and time it takes to find a husband. Dating other men and receiving phone calls from admirers usually doesn't go over too well with a live-in lover.

When you live with a guy for an extended period of time, you can become involved with his family and children (if any), and vice versa. Disentangling from these relationships can be a real source of conflict and turmoil. You may be close to and really care for some of his immediate relatives, and you may have grown accustomed to attending family gatherings, etc. This security may be one of your primary reasons for staying together. But if the family is as great as you believe them to be, then you can probably maintain a friendly, loving relationship with them . . . *after* you've kicked *him* to the curb. The longer you spend getting attached to him and his family, the harder it will be to extricate yourself from the situation. You're still expecting a high return on your initial investment. It may be difficult to do, but trust us—cut your losses and look for an entirely new game. Your odds are much better for long-term growth.

(Are you afraid of disrupting the "family" (kids, out-laws, social network)?   **Y N**

The bottom line is, you have to be willing to take some risks in order to secure your future happiness. Giving yourself time and space, a little pampering, and some reeducation (about the singles scene in your area, self-help groups, church or mosque, etc.) will take up plenty of time so that you won't feel too lonely or sad. Allowing yourself to grieve over what you once thought was a promising relationship will help fortify you for the future.

We feel the need to point out that some people do end up gettin' hitched after living together, but it's not the most direct route. If this ploy is so successful, why did you buy our book? (You know who you are . . .) We've found that getting him to marry you this way is like pulling teeth without any anesthetic. Do you really want to go through all of that pain and heartache? If you find yourself in that situation and you've already gone through a lot of pain and heartache, don't despair. Your emotional investment will pay off one day. You and only you can decide if your future is with this particular guy or not. Maybe, just maybe, he's not "The One." Or maybe he is, and you need to confront him. One day simply leave and see what happens.

Whatever the scenario, when it eventually happens, getting a proposal from the man of your dreams will be a very exciting moment in your life. It may not happen in the way you thought it would, but it *will* happen. You must think positively and believe that you are worthy of "all that and then some." Be communicative about your intentions and remain calm while you wait for your man to usher you into a different phase of your life as you make that mutual decision to marry.

Describe how you and your Black man decided to marry. Tell who proposed to whom and when.

_____

_____

_____

_____

_____

_____

_____

_____

_____

_____

_____

Was it like you imagined it would be? **Y N**

What did you say?

_____

_____

_____

_____

_____

What did he say?

_____

_____

_____

_____

Congratulations! We knew you could make it happen. Enjoy this moment of bliss 'cause the ride is just beginning. Get ready to plan a wedding. Here comes the Bride . . . !

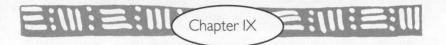
JuST Do It!

Word from the Brothahs

"I left it up to my wife, the wedding. And that's something that cost me $10,000."

"I want a big wedding...with lots of people and it's gonna cost a lot of money...because I know that's what my mother wants."

"Yes. I think I would enjoy something elaborate...whether it costs a lot or what it costs has nothing to do with it. It should be a celebration between two people."

"Does this mean that I love you less because our wedding cost $3,000 as opposed to $30,000?"

"I think they [womben] long to have a big wedding. It's like a fairy tale."

"A big wedding is gonna cost a lot of money."

"It can cost a lot of money or it can cost less than that. It just depends on how you do it. I mean, you can get someone with a big backyard and have a big wedding."

> "I was ecstatic with mine because I didn't spend any money."
>
> "When discussing the wedding and marriage, two people coming together, you don't want to come together on something that's gonna break you apart."
>
> "If you can spend $50,000 on a wedding and then get married and go buy a house, then okay, cool. Still, be able to afford it."
>
> "You only get married once. So she wants a big wedding, she gets a big wedding. Is that wrong?"
>
> "It's like if she wants to have a large wedding, you have to say, 'Listen, let me show you the bankbook. Let me tell you what's going on.'"
>
> "Some of my relatives complained not so much about *where* it was but what they had to *eat*."
>
> "You can't make two hundred people happy."

If only it was that simple. The unbelievable has happened! You're engaged to marry the man of your dreams. You now have the task of planning one of the most significant celebrations of your life: *your wedding!* We suggest that you try to have the wedding as soon as possible. We advise this for several reasons: The longer the engagement, the longer everyone has to drive you crazy . . . and they will. We guarantee it. The longer the engagement, the more time and money you have to spend. If you have a minimum of two months to plan the wedding, you won't have enough time to spend too much of either. Moreover, the sooner the wedding occurs the less time you or your groom have to get cold feet!

If you have children, you probably don't have time to plan a huge celebration. It takes a lot of ingenious planning to organize this very special event, and children can often zap your energy and ability to get things done.

Furthermore, we believe that too much significance is placed on the wedding ceremony when you plan a year ahead. All you do is dwell on costs and details of the events of one day instead of focusing on the incredible amount of tenacity and courage you'll need for a *forever* commitment.

And, finally, many of you are not spring chickens! Your biological clock is ticking! Why waste an entire year on an engagement when you could be incubating an egg? The sooner you get married, the sooner you can start that family you've always wanted.

Even if you don't want children, men change after the wedding (and you will too), so you might as well get used to the real thing as soon as possible. Because naturally the level of accommodation to each other will decrease and the level of compromise will increase. Why waste an entire year flirting with danger . . . just do it!

Unless you plan to elope, planning your wedding may be the first test of your relationship. The first thing you must realize is that this wedding is not really for the two of you. Weddings are for families and friends, not the bride and groom. With this in mind, you will quickly learn how important diplomacy is.

After he commits himself to the relationship and proposes, decide to get married by whatever means you both can afford and agree upon. Have open conversations about your expectations of your wedding ceremony. He doesn't want to disappoint you by not being able to give you the wedding of your dreams. He may also have some dreams himself, quiet as it's been kept. We've been brainwashed to believe that if we don't have a fairy-tale wedding, the marriage is doomed to failure. But we must remember what's really important. Our ancestors created intense tribal ceremonies to reinforce the idea that it's not about the bride and groom at all. In fact, the wedding ceremony served as the means by which the bride and groom were made aware that they were simply parts of a whole community and universe.

The Eurocentric traditions of spending huge amounts of money disregard the time-honored customs of creating a new family within the tribe. Paying strangers to handle all of the arrangements, while having our families attend as onlookers, may rob us of the true sharing of love and togetherness that's possible. Allowing everyone to do their share of cooking, decorating, costuming, flowering, and wording of a spiritual presentation solidifies the bride and groom's commitment to each other through witnessing the support from their extended families.

On the other hand, if you have the means with which to pull off nuptials more in line with the common trends and are willing to pay—yourself—for the events of one day, you'll have to massage his ego into accepting that it's okay to disregard the pressures from society, including the tribal community, that don't support a union between a "high-post gal" and a "low-post guy."

Bear in mind that his objections to the financial arrangement for the wedding may be the only way he knows to inform you that not only can he not afford such a wedding, but perhaps he has even more grave concerns that he can't handle an entire lifetime of financial inequality. Let's revive the old concept of the dowry. A womban comes into the marriage with money and the man has to take extremely good care of her and her resources, while still attempting to provide. The male ego can be quite fragile. And when it's directly connected to one of the few well-defined male role characteristics of being the bread winner, you must be extra careful about bruising his ego.

Before you tell anyone your wonderful news, you should start by sitting down with your intended to iron out a few things. *After* you decide on the very basics, you can tell your parents, family, and friends all about it.

Do both of you really want a wedding?	**Y N**
Is this the first time either of you is getting married?	**Y N**
If you are divorced, did you have a "Big Wedding" before?	**Y N**

If one of you was married before, perhaps neither of you really want a big deal again. However, this should not be a reason not to have a wedding ceremony. Don't give in to the feelings that because it didn't work out before, you don't deserve a celebration. It's strictly up to both of you.

How does he feel and think about it?

_____

_____

_____

How do you feel and think about it?

_____

_____

_____

Would you prefer to have a private, romantic civil ceremony? **Y** **N**

Do you want to have a religious ceremony? **Y** **N**

Do you belong to a church now? **Y** **N**

Some churches charge a nominal fee for a wedding. Usually, you must belong to the congregation or know a clergyman who belongs to that church. Do some investigating, call around, and get quotes from different places. You can always have the ceremony in a nontraditional location but still use a member of the clergy—you can have a religious ceremony in a park, by a lakeside, on a mountaintop, or aboard a boat. These are just a few of the places people have tied the knot.

Are you pregnant? **Y** **N**

Do you have children already? **Y** **N**

Do they approve of your intended? **Y** **N**

Does he have any children? **Y** **N**

Do they approve of you? **Y** **N**

Having a swift and efficient ceremony is always welcome if you are "with child," as they say. The longer you wait, the more you'll show. As the months go by, you'll grow more and more tired. Brides need their stamina. Try not to overexert yourself. Don't forget to pamper yourself—allow yourself lots of naps, and by all means rely on help from your intended. There won't be too many times in your lives together that you will need him more than you will right now! Lean on him, a lot!

If you or he already has children, they should be a primary consideration in your decision of whether or not to have a ceremony. Involving the children in the wedding ceremony is just the tip of the iceberg you'll be trying to melt as you try to blend the two families. Refer to Chapter X to rethink *all* of the issues involved. In some instances having a ceremony might be just what's needed to bring two families and traditions together. Then again, the children might use the wedding as a means to express their unhappiness at this new union by spoiling it completely. Anything is possible, so try to make sure you do the right thing for you and your fiancé first and then the children and families.

Reasons Not to Get Married

1. Just to be married. If you simply want to be coupled, just live together.
2. Wanting children. This is not a good reason to get married. Coparents are better than unhappy divorced parents. There isn't that basic hatred underlying the relationship. Having happy parents is much healthier for everyone involved. Don't let family pressure push you into something you're not ready for.
3. *Green Card* was a sweet movie, but... *hello!* Marrying an illegal alien so he can acquire American citizenship is a violation of immigration laws, a punishable federal offense. Hardly worth the money, time wasted, and aggravation. Besides, if you marry him for love and he's interested only in your status, you're cruising for an emotional bruising. But if the Brothah truly loves you... then go for it!

Can You Afford a Wedding?

Did your parents have a traditional "Big Wedding"?   **Y N**
Did his parents have a traditional "Big Wedding"?   **Y N**

If you answered "No" to one or both of the last two questions, be prepared for a hectic time. If your parents didn't have a wedding of their own, then they will likely be living out their wedding fantasies vicariously, through your nuptials. This is not necessarily bad, just be aware that they may have a hidden agenda. Let us not forget that traditionally the Mother of the Bride is responsible for the whole shebang! So remember this fact when your mother makes all of her loving but somewhat annoying suggestions. She is only doing what she thinks is expected of her.

What financial constraints exist?

_____

_____

Does your family approve of your intended?   **Y N**
Do you and/or your parents have the financial ability to pay
    for a wedding?   **Y N**

If your parents do not like your intended or just don't approve of your marrying him, be prepared to foot the bill alone or share expenses with your fiancé. More important, be prepared to face a lifetime of challenges without their support. If they express sincere rejection of your intended, it probably will last as long as he does. Can you tolerate nonsupport from your family for that long? Don't hedge your bets and assume that your family will come around. Prepare yourself for the worst. That way, if they do come around, so much the better. But if they don't, at least you're ready.

Do you have the ability to pay for a wedding? **Y N**
Does your intended have the ability to pay for a wedding? **Y N**
Do both of you together have the ability to pay for a wedding? **Y N**

If you answered "Yes" to any of the last questions, you should decide between yourselves who will take on the financial responsibility for the wedding.

How old are each of you? You _____ Him _____

Your age has a lot to do with deciding who will actually pay for the wedding. If you are a young couple, just starting out, and your families cannot afford to help you financially, then it might behoove you to have a civil ceremony and put your money toward a home or simply save it for the future. Remember that a large wedding ceremony does not make a successful marriage. We've witnessed many, many small, elegant, romantic ceremonies that get the job done without breaking the bank.

If you must make a fuss, there are ingenious ways to have wedding parties that don't cost an arm and a leg. If you know that you are not good at organizing such frugal events, call a friend or a family member who is. Ask your intended if he has a friend or family member who is good at making parties happen. Ask this person if he or she will help you plan and execute the wedding on a small budget. If you don't find the right person, then you'll have to take on the responsibility yourself. Make the wedding a family affair.

The secret is to get *everyone* in the two families involved. You must first survey all of the family members to find out who they are and what they have to offer. Then have a *family wedding*

planning meeting! Invite both families. Set an agenda of the tasks you need accomplished. The onus is on you to do all of the preplanning to determine exactly what is needed. Then explain what it is you want and how you plan to do it. Tell your family members what you are prepared to do yourself and then ask for help from each of them. Try to make all the family members feel as though they are being given a privilege instead of begged for their help. You will be surprised at how people enjoy joining in to assist a worthy cause. Remember that this often takes lots of creativity and dedication, but in the end you will be amazed at how successful your wedding will be.

Even if you do have the financial means to host a traditional wedding ceremony, having a family wedding planning meeting is still a great idea. Lots of times family members are capable of things that we have no idea they can do or have access to. If nothing else, ideas are just as valuable as money and resources, so get as many free ideas as possible. This meeting also will save you a lot of confusion and hurt feelings from family members who might otherwise feel slighted. As we said earlier, believe it or not, this wedding is more for them than for the two of you.

Pay special attention to the amount of involvement your groom has. The modern husband-to-be often wants equal input into all matters concerning the wedding, from bridal procession to honeymoon. If he wants to help in the planning, let him! If he is complaining that it seems to be "all about the womban," tell him that that's just the way it seems! Invite him to make as many suggestions as he wishes. It is, after all, his day too. You may be surprised—he just might have several great ideas to add.

If, on the other hand, you have a Groom who could care less about any of it, try to cultivate his interest by asking him lots and lots of specific questions. Usually this will spur him into asking a few questions of his own, if only "Why are you asking me so many questions?" That's when you take the opportunity to explain to him that planning something like this takes a great deal of forethought and his help is sorely needed.

Please be aware of two wedding (superstitious) traditions:

1. Do not show the groom your wedding dress/gown before the day of the wedding. Don't show him a photo of it, don't try it on for him, don't let him pick it up, and don't ask him if he likes it.

As far as we know it is considered *bad luck* to do any of the above. We're not quite sure where this superstition originated, but we have both witnessed cataclysmic results from brides ignoring this wedding superstition. The reason we decided to include this little tidbit of advice is that we feel it triggers other issues that a bride should consider before her wedding day, such as "Don't count you're chickens before they're hatched."

Superstitions and clichés aside, showing the groom your wedding ensemble prematurely displays a certain cockiness and manipulative ability that you may lord over him after you're married. As we pointed out earlier, men deplore any form of manipulation. So don't rub his nose in his newfound happiness, even if it is thanks to you, by jumping the gun.

2. On your Wedding Day wear something old, something new, something borrowed, and something blue.

Our mothers told us that their mothers told them. Why argue with that much wisdom? What can it hurt? It worked for us.

As for all of the other details you'll need to consider, we highly recommend *Jumping the Broom* by Harriette Cole as the quintessential African American wedding planner. She has captured the essence and beauty of an African American ceremony. Cole guides you through all of the necessary phases of planning a successful wedding with wonderful suggestions to make your wedding uniquely representative of our culture. *Jumping the Broom* serves as an etiquette guide as well. Cole makes it easy to "do the right thing" in every aspect of wedding planning. There are as many other wedding planning books on the market as there are brides. Check your local library and bookstores. You can create your own unique wedding by gleaning hints and tips from them all. The February issue of *Essence* always has a bridal feature, as it has for twenty-five years. The designs shown are generally Africentric, or at least inspired by other First World cultures. In any case, grab some books and magazines, get out your scissors, pad, and pen, and start planning!

Special note: We, as Black womben, must convince our Black Brothahs that marriage can be a sanctuary instead of a prison. We each have to recognize that we are capable of growth and development in our "spin" on the traditional Eurocentric view of marriage.

Create a fortress around your sanctuary of marriage so that he feels safe enough to confront his psychological demons. Make sure he knows that he can totally be himself and let all of his "warts" and "wounds" show in the confidentiality of your marriage. Encourage him to share his feelings, dreams, and fears with you. Cultivate an atmosphere of open communication and honesty. Help him to realize that there's nothing you can't discuss together and assure him that you would never judge him. Creating this fortress will be vital, not only to the survival of your marriage, but also for the continued growth of our race. Help him to help himself in the confidential sanctity of your own home. We feel having this marital sanctuary is a key factor in the Black man's strategy for continued success.

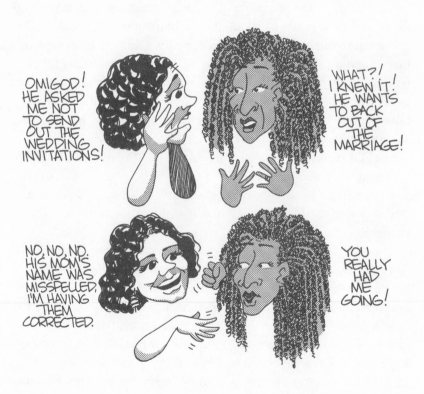

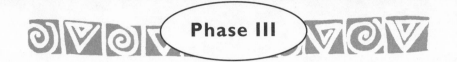

REAlITY cHECk

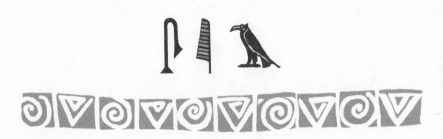

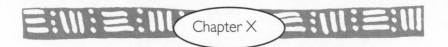

IF AT FIRST YOU DON'T SUCCEED . . .

"I got married again, for the cooking, for the companionship, for the support… but not for all the right reasons. I never really questioned what the right reasons were because I didn't even know who I was."

"My criteria now would be to find somebody who's not only compatible with me but somebody who truly respects me. I hear someone say compromising… but I think in a more giving of myself way… in order for it even to have a chance to work… because I always had to have it my way."

"Sometimes this person can leave you and that shows the most love for you… you know, if you're fuckin' up that bad. And that could still be unconditional love, because she may still love you but [is] doing what she has to do for herself… for *your* own good. So unconditional love doesn't mean letting you get away with everything. But it means she's still going to that love that you have in whatever action she has [to take]."

"When you date a Black womban that has a kid or two they're straight to the point, there's really no games played. They want to know which direction to go in and what your intention is. There's no charade."

"When you're involved with someone and you do shit that really hurts that person, it changes you, you know?"

If at first you don't succeed . . . Forget about it! Why would you want to get hooked again anyway? You see that it didn't work out the first time. You can have companionship, friendship, partnership, sex, and even kids without the benefit of marriage, so what's the point?

Whether you've been married or in a long-term, serious relationship, read this chapter. If you're thinking about taking that awesome step again, take time to investigate why the first union didn't work. "You'd better check yourself before you wreck yourself!" Face the facts. You have some baggage you need to get rid of, or at least own up to.

In your former marriage(s), where were the points of contention?

_____

_____

_____

What part did you play in the dissolution of your previous marriage(s)?

_____

_____

_____

Have you accepted responsibility for your part? **Y N**

Have you forgiven yourself for your part? **Y N**

What part did your former husband play in the dissolution of your previous marriage(s)?

_____

_____

_____

_____

Has he accepted responsibility for his part? **Y N**

Has he apologized? **Y N**

Have you apologized? **Y N**

Have you expressed your underlying hurt and anger directly
   to him and/or to family and friends or a counselor? **Y N**

Have you forgiven him? **Y N**

Should you forgive him? **Y N**

If he has not apologized, can you forgive him anyway, for
   your own sake? **Y N**

Hopefully, you've recognized that you both played major roles in the breakup of your relationship. Acknowledgment of your part has allowed you to forgive yourself and move on. You also have to face the fact that, for whatever reason, he doesn't want to be in a relationship with you anymore. You must confront your former mate with your anger, hurt, and disappointment before you can forgive him. It might not be possible to confront him in person because he might have died or moved far away. Write a letter expressing your anger and frustration or role-play with a friend or counselor. Even if there has been physical or mental abuse, it helps *you* to forgive the person, not the behavior.

Note: If you have removed yourself from any kind of violently abusive situation, you will have to do your confrontation through group therapy or counseling. Do not put yourself in physical danger.

On some level, you will always be connected to this man, especially if you have children. The phrase "till death do you part" resonates in your heart and soul. But think about all the little deaths you have mourned throughout the demise of your relationship. They each add up to a point where you realize that, for all intents and purposes, the man you married is "dead." If you're a widow, you must allow yourself to grieve in the best way you know how (see vow on p. 47). This private process of healing is more than necessary so that you can go on with your life—it's crucial for your future happiness. After a significant period of time, you will be able to love another.

You cannot move into a mature, healthy relationship until and unless you have done this work and mourned the death of your marriage. If you have, according to the vows you made, you release yourself to move on to something else.

How do you feel about your wedding vows now?

_____

_____

Are you able to keep that commitment this time? Seriously?

_____

_____

How can you be sure?

_____

_____

How will you change or adapt your wedding vows the next time around?

_____

_____

_____

_____

You may be asking what the difference is between a divorce and the breakup of a long-term, serious relationship. Sometimes there's not much difference at all. Don't avoid dating someone because you suspect that he's not "The One." We all learn things about ourselves through each relationship we have. The secret is to try to not make the same mistakes over, and over, and over again, but to learn *new* lessons with each encounter.

Rebound Relationships, for instance, serve an important purpose. They can help you to heal and regain some of the nurturing you may have missed out on in your previous relationship(s). The imperative thing to remember about rebounding is that sometimes we try to fool ourselves, and try to substitute them for the real thing. This usually doesn't last long. Reality always wins out.

Look at what you've gained from this encounter with this person. What have you learned about yourself?

_____

_____

_____

_____

_____

What have you gotten out of knowing this person?

_____

_____

_____

_____

We all go through periods of learning about ourselves through painful, sometimes heartbreaking experiences. They only make us stronger and more sure of the things we need and want, so that when "He" does come along, we're ready for him!

How Ya Livin'?

Look at your life right now. Describe a "typical" day.

_____

_____

_____

_____

_____

In the typical day that you described:

Was there time for you and you alone?	**Y N**
Did you have a relaxing bath?	**Y N**
Did you meditate for fifteen minutes to an hour?	**Y N**
Did you write in your journal?	**Y N**
Did you spend an hour reading?	**Y N**
Did you do something just for you?	**Y N**

If you answered "No" to three or more questions, then you don't have the psychic space needed to include a mate in your life right now. You need to have regular private time for reflection, relaxation, and rejuvenation. You *should* have it every day, but at the least every other day, not just once a week or once a month, in order to maintain some semblance of sanity.

If you work, is it a job or a career? _____

Many of us spend much of our waking time committed to
someone else's goals and aspirations. In your Five-Year Plan,
did you map out career plans?   **Y N**

If not, do so now.

_____

_____

_____

_____

_____

If you're happy in your work, it will feed and fulfill you. Unhappy work situations are draining and frustrating, and they leave you depleted so that you don't have the time or energy to focus on your own life. Of course, we realize that there are practical reasons that necessitate staying in certain types of jobs: keeping a roof over your head, feeding yourself and your kids, maintaining health insurance, and the like. We simply encourage you to find ways to improve your situation by going back to school, getting onto a career track, finding a job that is fulfilling, or maybe even starting your own business. If you want to find out more about how to determine what your new career path should be, we highly recommend purchasing the most recent edition of *What Color Is Your Parachute: A Practical Manual for Job-Hunters and Career-Changers* by Richard Nelson Bolles.

The Dating Game

Being a divorcée can be exhilarating. The sense of freedom and limitless opportunities can be both exciting and frightening. You probably looked at your options before you made the final decision to divorce—unless, of course, you were in an abusive relationship and didn't think the possibility existed for you. But if you're reading this book, you're probably ready to go!

If you don't have kids, skip the next section (and come back to it when you have kids or start dating a guy who does). As you may have found out by now, kids can destroy a relationship even before it starts, especially if you let them.

Friends for the Sake of the Kids

What kind of relationship do you have with your child(ren)'s father(s)?

____ Friendly

____ Hostile

____ Communicative

_____ Third-party-mediated
_____ Nonexistent

I would not resent my partner's contact with
  His former wife   **Y N**
  His child(ren)'s mother   **Y N**
  His former lover   **Y N**
I would encourage my partner's child(ren) to talk about their
  mother.   **Y N**

Having a good relationship with your former partner allows you to recognize and respect _his_ previous relationships with womben who may also have children by him. It might be easier for you to embrace this concept if you think of it as another, more modern aspect of the extended family.

It can be very difficult after breaking up with someone to re-create a friendship with him, but if you share parenthood with that person, it is essential. The children will be happier. If Mommy and Daddy get along, there is less chance that they will feel compelled to take sides or blame themselves. It might also facilitate good relationships with your former partner's family, which widens your support network. So why cut off your nose to spite your face? While the children are young, you are proba-bly going to have to take on the responsibility of outreach to and communication with their father.

Many of you have had terrible experiences with your chil-dren's father(s). You feel that there is no way on earth that you will ever be friends with this man again. But put yourself in your child's place. You, the child, love both of these people, but they hate each other. If you have a problem with one of them, you can't go to the other to help you figure it out. As a parent, you want to give your child every opportunity to learn and grow in a healthy way. Don't put down the child's father. If he truly is a jerk, sooner or later the child will figure it out on his or her own. Your job is simply to provide the space for that to happen naturally.

Another aspect to keeping, renewing, or developing a friendship with your children's father is that of maintaining the children's routine. Isn't it better for the children to have similar rules and situations with both parents than to have totally opposite environments to operate in? This consistency is not possible if you're not communicating with each other.

A commonly accepted reason for not being friendly with your children's father is his sporadic or complete lack of child support payments. Let that be a separate issue, apart from the issue of parental support. We acknowledge that this may be one of the hardest things that you'll ever do, but it is major. Maintain a civil relationship with him, and let the lawyers, social workers, or mediators handle the rest. You don't have to be the guy's best friend, just be cordial enough to elicit the children's respect for him as their father. After all, if he's done nothing else, he's helped to give them life.

Although differing childrearing strategies may have been one of your points of conflict while you were together, you had to compromise. Try to keep that sensibility operating. Conversely, if you are still sleeping with the guy, you have a different situation to evaluate. You must find a way to convert your safe, familiar sexual haven into a familiar parental haven for your children. Remember that we advise all women to abstain from sex for a certain amount of time if they are thinking of remarrying. This applies doubly to you because it just isn't healthy to keep opening that part of yourself to a man who is no longer committed to you. At the very least, help him stay committed to your children. They will prosper and grow from his regular input and caring. As an added bonus, you can use the times they are with him for your own purposes, especially dating.

Are you currently dating anyone?   **Y N**
Are there any children involved?   **Y N**
On either or both sides?   **E B**

If you have kids, what are your custodial arrangements?
Joint custody _____   Sole custody _____   Visitation rights _____

Are you receiving or paying child support?   **R P**

If he has kids, what are his custodial arrangements?
Joint custody _____   Sole custody _____   Visitation rights _____

Is he receiving or paying child support?   **R P**

Your responsibility to your children is to make sure that they are sufficiently fed and housed. It doesn't matter if you are receiving child support. Not that it isn't important for their father to live up to his responsibility to them, but it may not be something that you can rely on through the years. God bless the child that's got his own.

This is a good reason to try to be self-sufficient financially. You don't want to be dependent on a future mate who may have child support issues of his own. Don't allow yourself to waver from this position until you've been convinced that your future husband sincerely intends to share support for *all* children equally.

Children go through *different* phases as they grow. It is important to remember that you understand them much better than your new partner.

Are your kids

Outgoing?	**Y N**
Shy?	**Y N**
Well adjusted?	**Y N**
Close to their dad?	**Y N**
Independent?	**Y N**
Well disciplined?	**Y N**
Doing well in school?	**Y N**
"Special needs" kids?	**Y N**
On a schedule for bedtimes, meals, and homework?	**Y N**

You need to discuss these aspects of your children's lives with your mate.

Can he deal with your kids? **Y N**

Regular homework and mealtimes not only give the kids a sense of stability but also allow you to spend quality time with them. Regular bedtimes give you "down time" with peace and quiet in your own home. You might also be able to sneak in a late date here and there. Despite the kids, you can still have an active sexual life with prospective mates. A good way to do this is to either have the kids spend the night out or make sure they are asleep by the time you return home with your date. Equally important is to make sure that your date's up and out before the kids wake up. It can be helpful to have a latch on your bedroom door to ensure privacy throughout the night, especially if your kids have a tendency to awaken at inopportune times.

By not immediately involving the children in your relationships with new men, you can survey a few candidates without exposing your kids to emotional interactions that they may come to depend on.

Do you immediately tell the men you're dating that you have
   children?   **Y N**
Do you wait until you think he's ready for a serious,
   committed relationship?   **Y N**

Be open about your children and their needs with prospective mates, right from the start. If you have children, give him the chance to decide whether or not he wants to continue your relationship. It can only help you to focus on what your needs are for yourself, your children, and your future mate.

Do you have on-call, overnight child care available?   **Y N**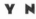

What are your child-care arrangements when you have a date?

_____

_____

Good reliable child care is hard to find, but it is possible. Networking with other mothers who have the same age kids, your former husband or his family members, your family members, etc., can help you get out there and get a life again.

Another issue that must be dealt with delicately and diplomatically is the spiritual path that you and your children are on. If you're not on any particular spiritual path with your children, then you should take some time now to plan for their spiritual upbringing. If the children are at an age of awareness, include them in conversations about spirituality. If you are already well grounded in your spirituality, determine how important continuing your current path is to you. Try to evaluate your openness to change or compromise, in case your future mate is on a different path and plan to communicate some of your thoughts to him.

What spiritual path are you and your family on now?

_____

_____

Assessing Your Readiness to Try Again

Now that you've gotten your life together as a single parent and are ready for a serious commitment, are you prepared to see your life change? Go ahead and get married again! After you've met someone and you're dating seriously, but before you actually get married and attempt to blend your two families into one, consider this: It is guaranteed that at the beginning, *everyone in-*

volved will have problems and complaints and will find someone or something irritating.

The best way to deal with these problems is to encourage the expression of and listen to each individual's complaints. Discuss the problems with your future mate and make sure you present a united front to the children. This is crucial.

Here are some questions to make you think about some of the situations you will face and the problem solving required in blending families. When you find a prospective mate, make sure he answers these questions too.

I expect the children to

Respect me **Y N**

Obey me **Y N**

Love me **Y N**

Are you prepared to give a lot to stepchildren and get little
or nothing in return? **Y N**

I discipline children by

Listening **Y N**

Talking **Y N**

Screaming/yelling **Y N**

Spanking/beating **Y N**

Punishment **Y N**

All of the above **Y N**

Children should be disciplined by

Me **Y N**

My partner **Y N**

Both **Y N**

If my mate engages in a serious conflict with my child, I expect to
_____ Reinforce his authority   _____ Challenge his authority

I will grant him
_____ Complete authority   _____ Limited authority

The way I handle children is
_____ Authoritarian   _____ Submissive
_____ Flexible   _____ Rigid
_____ Kind   _____ Harsh
_____ Understanding   _____ Intolerant

The way my partner handles children is
_____ Authoritarian   _____ Submissive
_____ Flexible   _____ Rigid
_____ Kind   _____ Harsh
_____ Understanding   _____ Intolerant

When there is a conflict between my mate and my child, my mate
   should
_____ Come up with a compromise
_____ Consult me
_____ Ignore it and let it blow over

My children's other parent wants to change custody
   arrangements. I would
_____ Be happy to change them
_____ Expect to be consulted
_____ Refuse to consider it
_____ Fight it tooth and nail

My mate or my mate's children's other parent wants to change custody arrangements. I would

_____ Not care if they change

_____ Expect to be consulted

_____ Refuse to consider it

_____ Fight it tooth and nail

I expect my mate to provide financially for me and my children. **Y N**

Children should participate in household chores. **Y N**

Household chores are the responsibility of

Me **Y N**

My partner **Y N**

Both **Y N**

Children should participate with me and my mate in

_____ All social activities   _____ Most social activities

_____ Some social activities   _____ No social activities

Holiday traditions are important. My favorite/most important holidays and traditions are

_____

_____

Children should be present and/or participate in certain customs and family traditions. They are

_____

_____

I would like to vacation

_____ Alone   _____ With my mate

_____ With the children   _____ With the whole family

_____ Sometimes with the children and sometimes without

As a coparent, the most important thing I can do for my mate after we marry will be

_____

_____

_____

The Name Game

When you remarry, you must consider your new name and the name(s) of your children. After you divorced, did you revert to your maiden name or did you keep your married name?   _____

How do you think you'll handle this issue when you remarry?

_____

_____

_____

Think about how your children will feel at school or on other occasions when they'll have to introduce you as "My mom, Mrs. So-and-So. Consider the situation if you were to have more children. Will they bear your name? His name? Some combination of the two? These are some of the things you must consider.

Another aspect of remarrying with children is that of adoption.

Would you want your future husband to adopt your children? **Y N**
Would your children want to be adopted? **Y N**
Do the ages of the children affect your decision? **Y N**
Would the costs of legal fees deter you? **Y N**
Would the wishes of the children's father affect you? **Y N**

How do you think adoption would affect your children's relationship with their father?

_____

_____

_____

_____

_____

Adoption is a serious and delicate issue. The ages of the children, their relationship with their father, their relationship with your future husband, and many other important issues must be considered. If the children are very young or don't have a close relationship with their father, the decision might be a little easier. Older children who already have attachments to their father or who have decided that they don't like your choice of a new mate may present a problem. Don't rush into anything. Take your time to discuss with your mate, your children, and the children's father all the issues that will influence your decision. Research the legal ramifications. There may be legal reasons that you won't want to consider adoption for your children. Whatever you decide to do, make sure it's the best choice for you and your children.

We are not trying to focus on the negative aspects of blending families, but on the gritty realities. Yes, the questions we've posed are difficult, but what you are about to embark on is much more difficult than answering them. Forewarned is forearmed.

You must first do all of the required healing in order to go on with your life. We hope the meditations in Chapter II have helped you to grow stronger. You have to sort out *all* of these things before you remarry. The stakes may seem higher to you, and you may be a little wary. This is perfectly understandable. Try not to be disillusioned or too set in your ways. Leave the bitterness pill for someone else to take. Whether you're divorced or you've been abandoned or widowed, your kids are going to grow and leave you alone as they continue with their own lives. So you must consider your own needs and feelings and realize that it is perfectly all right to make them a priority.

A second marriage can be one of the most rewarding relationships you'll ever have, but you should look long and hard at your motivation before jumping in again.

Be careful what you ask for. You might get it. Next time, make sure you're ready.

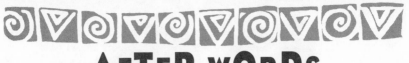

AfTeR wORDs

FOOD FOR THOUGHT

Word from the Brothahs

"I think for a relationship to work on the level of marriage, both people have to be willing to be completely, totally, utterly vulnerable to each other. I mean, I want to be able to see my womban at her lowest of lows and still say in my head, 'Damn, I still love this womban!'

"I don't want to have to continually be prideful and dignified in front of my womban because I have enough of that in the outside world. Elements such as pride, ego, and dignity can really destroy a relationship...and I just want to be able to be totally, totally vulnerable in front of my womban, you know, at my ugliest, my weakest, my lowest of lows...and have that person still look at me and say 'Damn, I love this man.' If I could find a womban who could love me on that level, then I'd be ready to get married in a minute. One minute!"

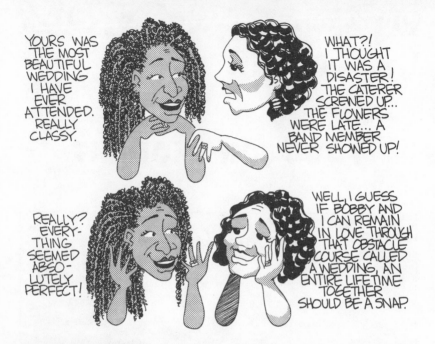

Wow!! You've made it to the end of the book! Congratulations! Do you think that you have followed the program successfully? We know that you have the power! You've made some empowering choices and monumental decisions.

What are some of the changes you've made so far?

_____

_____

_____

Much of what you've gone through in the process of using this book has been self-evaluation and reevaluation. You should now know more about yourself than you ever have before.

What are some of the things you've discovered about yourself?

_____

_____

_____

_____

_____

Take this knowledge and fly! Read like you've never read before. The suggested reading list at the back of the book will get you started. Remember, you can come back to this book at any time. Hopefully, it will be a source of information and comfort for you, a tool that will help you sort things out and get focused.

Marriage is one of the greatest challenges you will ever face. You will grow through shared experiences with a friend. Your spiritual, emotional, intellectual, and social growth may astound you. Through love and communication, your two lives can become one greater life, enhancing the parts that combine to form the whole.

Now, go back to the beginning and fill in all those exercises that you skipped. Can't do no half-stepping now, Sis! Peace.

Life Partners

Our spirits fly through the universe to join in a joyous union

That comforts us in spite of the distance of our uniqueness

I want to hold you,

wrap my arms around you,

whisper sweet somethings in your ear.

Lick your lips, kiss your eyebrows.

Taste your nectar.

This hunger I feel for you has taken away my appetite for bodily

nourishment.

I melt at the thought of being near you,

at the touch of your hand on mine,

at the sound of your rough voice.

Feed my hungry body.

Quench the thirst of my desire with your mere presence.

Satiate my spirit with sustenance from your soul,

Your body touches mine,

y s

g e

r s

e i

n R

E

We come together

In mind, body, soul, and spirit.

Hands and hearts entwined by love.

I want to promise you the moon...the stars...a galaxy of love,

I can only give you my Self...

Today...tomorrow and

Tomorrow...and tomorrow...

I look into your eyes and see reflected my beauty,

my love,

my sweetness,

and my light,

that grow with each passing day.

Your gentle acceptance enables me to thrive,

To approach the tempting vistas my soul yearns to explore,

Vast horizons beckon endlessly...

Yet my connection to you is solidly ephemeral.

As is the silver cord that binds this body

to that ceaselessly searching soul.

Stay with me.

Let us share our joys, our sorrows, our feelings.

Let nothing that comes between us separate us.

Our belief in our fidelity allows us to remain in a state of bliss,

The seldom found condition that binds two lives...

together...

eternally...

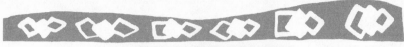

MO' STUFF

GLOSSARY OF SLANGUAGE

We've included this dictionary to keep you up-to-date with the current *Black talk* in our community. Don't feel bad if you're not familiar with some of the phrases and words that are sprinkled throughout the book. Just look up anything you don't get. We are proud of the innovative oral tradition that makes everyday conversations in the *'hood* stimulating and comforting. This reworking of English reassures us that we *do* influence popular culture—*big time!*—and that this influence is rooted in the knowledge that "It's a Black thang, you wouldn't understand!"

Most of the words we've used have been popular for decades. Some of the old words, like *hip*, are beginning to reemerge with a youthful spin. Black English, as has been documented, is a combination of traditional African words, concepts, and pronunciations. Some of the other words and phrases we define are not exactly *slanguage*, but they may be unfamiliar to you. You might use different expressions in your area. If there's something that you've never heard of before or can't find in any other slang dictionary, don't worry, we probably made it up on the spot!

Peace out.

About; about too much: See Be(in') 'bout.

Ad-dick-tive: Capable of causing fixation on the dick.

Ad-venture: Experience resulting from reading/answering a personal ad.

Ain't all that (much): Not measuring up to one's standards.

All that, all that (much) and then some (more): Excellent; gorgeous; magnificent; fine.

All the way live: Occurrence taking place in one's presence; exciting; original happening that is not prerecorded.

A'wastin': Wasting.

Back: Loyalty or protection no matter what the consequences; butt. See *also* Have your back.

Back up off of: Slow down (as a romantic pursuit).

Back up on some of your stuff: Compromise; reevaluate your position.

Bag a brothah: Get a Black man to marry you.

Baggin': The act of getting a Black man into marriage or a serious relationship.

Beating the bushes: Searching tirelessly; making a concerted effort to find something.

Be doggin': Treating poorly; neglecting.

Be(in') 'bout: Being involved in doing something meaningful.

Big dipper: Penis.

Big time: Extremely.

Black butterfly: Black man who is artistic or musically inclined.

Black talk: African American's adaptation of European language; Black English.

Bounty hunter: A family member, friend, or associate who is looking for a husband for you; matchmaker.

Boyz: Boys; men.

Brothah: Brother.

Brown sugar: A sexy, sweet, brown-skinned person; the love received from that person, especially sexual.

Buppie: Black Urban Professional.

Case of the ass: Attitude of negativity; state of being irritated, sometimes without a discernible cause.

Chakra: Powerful spiritual centers (spirals) of energy found in certain locations throughout the body (from Eastern spiritual traditions).

Check yourself before you wreck yourself: Acknowledge and change negative behavior before it's too late; think about actions before heading into a disaster.

Children of the rainbow: Offspring from interracial unions; gay people.

Chill: Sit back and relax: *See also* Cool.

Chucklehead: Idiot, fathead.

Clue you: Give you a hint as to what is actually going on.

Cool: Relaxed.

Coparents: People who commit financially, legally, morally, and physically to conceive and/or adopt a child to raise together.

Cozy Coo: Comfortable.

Darfore: Therefore.

Dat: That.

Def: (*From* death) serious.

Dis: Short for disrespect or dismiss.

Diva: Womban who either is glamorous or puts on airs of glamour.

Dog: Man who has random, casual, sexual relationships, like a dog; man who uses romance and sex to manipulate wombens for ulterior purposes and/or money.

Doggin': Treating poorly, like a dog.

Do me (any) justice: Give me what I deserve, what's fair.

Don't go there: Don't entertain the notion; don't consider whatever it is you're considering; refrain from even thinking about certain topics.

Do shit: Accomplish things.

Fantasies on tap: Daydreams or illusions that one usually thinks about, especially sexual.

Faze: Bother, move.

Feel-think: Person who responds by considering emotions before thinking things through: *See also* Think-feel.

Fierce: Sharp; tough.

Fine: Handsome; sexy.

First World: Formerly known as Third World; all African, Latin American, and so-called underdeveloped countries.

Foreplay letter: Note that suggests erotic possibilities and/or fantasies.

Four-one-one (411): Information; gossip.

Fo'word: Foreword of a book.

From the get-go: From the very beginning.

Fronting: Putting up a false facade; covering up.

Fuck-buddy: Friend with whom one has sex when horny; someone with whom one has little or no emotional attachment. *See also* Insertable man; Maintenance man.
Fugitive: Man who is commitment-phobic.

Gazillion: Uncountable number: *See also* Umpteenmillion.
Geared up: Dressed up.
Get a clue: Become aware of a situation.
Get a grip: Get control of oneself or a situation.
Get over it: Release whatever *it* is.
Get the cash and dash: Take the money and run.
Gigging: Working.
Girlfriend: Womban.
Girlz: Womben.
Giving head: Performing oral sex.
Giving out the signals: Sending a nonverbal communication; especially of readiness for marriage.
Givin' the 411: Providing the information; gossiping.
Go down on: Perform oral sex on (male or female).

Half-steppin': Not making a full or complete effort.
Handyman: Great guy who is helpful and loving.
Happin'n'; Happenin': Current and enjoyable.
Have your back: Watching out for your best interests; providing protection.
Herstory: History as it relates to womben.
Hip: Up-to-date.
'Hood: Neighborhood.
Hook up: Meet; become steady dates; get together with; marry: *See also* Jumping the broom.
Hot: Contemporary; intensely sexual; great. *See also* Fierce.
House party: Function given at someone's home.

I.M.: Instant message.
In a big way: With great enthusiasm.
Insertable man/womban: Partner of convenience available for certain occasions.
Into: Focused on; liking.

Jam: Joyous celebration; impromptu musical improvisation; have sex.
Jazz up: Upgrade; spruce up; spice up.

Jibe: Blend; fit together.

Jive: Not serious or committed; deceitful.

Jump the broom: Get married.

Jungle fever: Attraction between a Black person and a white person.

Keep on the hook: Keep someone interested.

Kickin' (him) to the curb: Getting rid of (him).

Little red book:: Small telephone book with numbers of hot prospects, hence the color red.

Long haul: Extended period of time.

Lube: Non-petroleum-based lubrication jelly used to facilitate sexual intercourse.

Maintenance man: A man whose primary purpose in one's life is sexual; *See also* Fuck-buddy; Insertable man/womban.

Mission: Focused drive; usually used in speaking of sex or drugs.

Motherland: Africa.

Mother wit: Intuition; common sense; street smarts.

M word: Marriage.

Name game: Process of picking a new family name once married; what one must play when remarrying, especially as it relates to children.

Nitty Gritty: Undiplomatic version of the facts; central issues; heart of the matter.

No-back-out clause: Agreement to stay till death do you part; marriage.

On a mission: Being single-minded about getting something (done); *See also* Mission.

On tap: On hand; at the ready; lined up.

Opened the circuit: Made some mental connections.

Out-laws: Family who would be related after marriage; once in-laws by marriage, now out-laws after divorce; premarital relatives.

Papi: Term of endearment.

Par-tay: Party; Have a really good time.

Peace out: Good-bye.

Perfect stranger: Man who seems to be extremely likely candidate on first meeting.

Phat: Fat; really great; excellent; superb.

Piece of (wedding) cake: Easy.

Pink bubble man: Man one creates in the imagination using all of the parts of old boyfriends/lovers, as well as desired personality traits, class, and financial status, husband to be.

Play: Use and/or abuse.

Play you: Manipulate you in such a way that you are being made to look and/or act like a fool.

Plumbing: Sexual organs.

Pretty boy: Stylish, handsome guy; looker.

Private dancer: Someone who dances for or with one person; reference to a Tina Turner song about dancing for one.

Promise ring: Token of commitment.

Rags: Clothes.

Real deal: Authentic; honest facts.

Reality check: Comparison of perceived information and actual facts; reassessment of life or a situation.

Red-hot number: Number of a prospective man newly met: See *also* Little red book.

Risky business: Something having an uncertain outcome; taking a tremendous chance.

Rusty: Unused; out of practice.

Safe house: Place in which to hide or be protected.

Safer sex: Limiting the exchange of bodily fluids during foreplay or sexual intercourse through the use of latex barriers, especially condoms (male or female) and dental dams.

Scoping: Viewing; looking at.

Screwing: Having sex.

Sistah: Black womban.

Sistah under the skin: Close sibling-like friendship regardless of race.

Slammin' time: Great experience.

Slanguage: Modern Black English.

Smooth talker: One who is able to converse easily on many subjects.

Snap: Easy; simple; a put-down.

Socking away extra change: Saving money.

Soul searching: Looking deeply inside oneself.

Squat: Shit; nothing.

Strapped for cash: Condition when money is tight or hard to come by; broke.

Sugah: Someone or something sweet: See *also* Brown sugar.

Surfin' the net: Goin on-line to observe situations and discover new information.

Take: Interpretation.

Talkin' that talk: Using Black English dynamically, energetically, intensely, and correctly.

Thang: Thing.

The Man: The white man; the boss; a drug dealer; the police.

The One: Man one will marry.

Them's the breaks: That's the way things happen.

Think-feel: Person who responds by thinking through before considering emotions: *See also* Feel-think.

Throwing the jam: Hosting a party.

Tip off: Make aware of.

Togedder: See togethah.

Togethah: In order; correct; well thought-out; everything in place; ready.

Trademark: Distinguishing or outstanding characteristic.

Trap: Compel into a situation that one can't escape.

Tribe: Group with whom one has an affinity.

Umpteenmillion: I-don't-know-how-many million times; more than one would care to name. *See also* Gazillion.

Waiting to pounce: Anticipating the moment.

What time it is: The real situation.

Where (one's) head was at: What or how one was thinking.

Whole shebang: Everything; all plans.

Wild thang: Sexual intercourse.

Womban: Adult female.

Word: Affirmative.

Yo': Your.

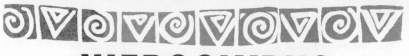

HIEROGLYPHS

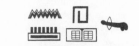

Wisdom

Marriage, Consummation

Recognize, Know, Understand

Writing, Book

Heart

RECOMMENDED READING

Emotional

Estes, Clarissa P. *Women Who Run with the Wolves: Myths and Stories of the Wild Women Archetype*. New York: Ballantine, 1995.

Evans, Patricia, *Verbal Abuse Survivors Speak Out: On Relationship and Recovery*. Holbrook, Mass.: Bob Adams, 1993.

Fassler, David, Michelle Lash, and Sally Blakeslee Ives. *Changing Families: A Guide for Kids and Grown-ups*. Burlington, VT.: Waterfront Books, 1988.

Fregia, Pat and Jim. *Know Your Dreams: Know Your Self: A Workbook*. Berkeley, Calif.: Celestial Arts, 1994.

Hansen Shaevitz, Marjorie. *The Superwoman Syndrome*. New York: Warner Books, 1984.

Hill, Ivan. *The Bisexual Spouse: Different Dimensions in Human Sexuality*. New York: Perennial Library/Harper & Row, 1989.

Keyes, Ken, and Penny Keyes. *The Power of Unconditional Love: Twenty-one Guidelines for Beginning, Improving, and Changing Your Most Meaningful Relationships*. Coos Bay, Oreg.: Love Line Books, 1990.

Kiley, Dr. Dan. *Living Together, Feeling Alone: Healing Your Hidden Loneliness*. New York: Prentice Hall, 1989.

Lerner, Goldhor Harriet, Ph.D. *The Dance of Intimacy: A Woman's Guide to Courageous Acts of Change in Key Relationships*. New York: Harper & Row, 1989.

Middleton-Moz, Jane. *Children of Trauma: Rediscovering the Discarded Self*. Deerfield Beach, Fla.: Health Communications, 1989.

Norwood, Robin. *Women Who Love Too Much: When You Keep Wishing and Hoping He'll Change*. New York: Pocket Books, 1986.

Scarf, Maggie. *Intimate Partners: Patterns in Love and Marriage*. New York: Ballantine Books, 1988.

Smith, Manuel. *When I Say No I Feel Guilty*. New York: Simon & Schuster, 1987.

Spiritual

Andrews, Lynn. *Medicine Woman.* New York: Perennial Library, 1981.

Castaneda, Carlos. *The Teachings of Don Juan: A Yaqui Way of Knowledge.* Berkeley, Calif.: University of California Press, 1968.

Ozaniiec, Naomi. *The Elements of the Chakras.* Shaftesbury, Dorset/Rockport, Mass.: Element Books, 1990.

Redfield, James. *The Celestine Prophecy.* New York: Warner Books, 1993.

Sjoo, Monica, and Barbara Mor. *The Great Cosmic Mother: Rediscovering the Religion of the Earth.* San Francisco: Harper & Row, 1987.

Teish, Luisa. *Jambalaya: The Natural Woman's Book of Personal Charms and Practical Rituals.* San Francisco: Harper & Row, 1985.

Van Zant, Iyanla. *Acts of Faith: Daily Meditations for People of Color.* New York: Fireside/Simon & Schuster, 1993.

Walker, Barbara G. *The Women's Encyclopedia of Myths and Secrets.* San Francisco: Harper & Row, 1983.

Physical

Boston Women's Collective. *The New Our Bodies Ourselves: A Book by and for Women.* New York: Simon & Schuster, 1984.

Cornish, Gracie. *Radiant Women of Color.* New York: Kola Publishing, 1994.

Gregory, Richard. *Dick Gregory's Natural Diet for Folks Who Eat: Cookin' with Mother Nature.* New York: Harper & Row, 1973.

Hittleman, Richard, *Richard Hittleman's Yoga: Twenty-eight-Day Exercise Plan.* New York: Bantam, 1967, 1982.

Villarosa, Linda, ed. *Body and Soul: The Black Woman's Guide to Physical Health and Emotional Well-being.* New York: HarperCollins, 1994.

Wolf, Naomi. *The Beauty Myth: How Images of Beauty Are Used Against Women.* New York: Morrow, 1991.

Youcha, Geraldine. *Women and Alcohol: A Dangerous Pleasure.* New York: Crown, 1986.

Sexual

Anand, Margo. *The Art of Sexual Ecstasy: The Path of Sacred Sexuality for Western Lovers.* Los Angeles: J. P. Tarcher, 1989.

Chia, Mantak, and Maneewan Chia. *Healing Love Through the Tao: Cultivating Female Sexual Energy.* Huntington, N.Y.: Healing Tao Books, 1986.

Comfort, Alex. *The New Joy of Sex.* New York: Crown, 1991.

Decosta-Willis, Reginald Martin, and Roseann P. Bell. *Erotique Noire: Black Erotica.* New York: Anchor/Doubleday. 1993.

Love, Patricia, and Jo Robinson. *Hot Monogamy: Essential Steps to More Passionate, Intimate Lovemaking.* New York: Dutton, 1994.

Cultural

Anzaldua, Gloria. *Making Face, Making Soul: Haciendo Caras, Creative and Critical Perspectives by Women of Color.* San Francisco: Aunt Lute Books, 1990.

Asante, Molefi K. *Afrocentricity.* Trenton, N.J.: Africa World Press, 1988.

————. *New Dimensions in African History: The London Lectures of Dr. Yosef Ben-Jochannan and Dr. John Henrik Clarke.* Trenton, N.J.: Africa World Press, 1991.

Crohn, Joel. *Mixed Matches: How to Create Successful Interracial, Interethnic, Interfaith Relationships.* New York: Fawcett Columbine, 1995.

Davis, Angela. *Women, Culture, and Politics.* New York: Vintage Books, 1990.

Diop, Cheikh Anta. *Civilization or Barbarism: An Authentic Anthropology.* N.Y.: Lawrence Hill Books, 1991.

Gates, Henry Louis, ed. *Reading Black, Reading Feminist: A Critical Anthology.* New York: Meridan Books, 1990.

Gilbert, Olive. *Narrative of Sojourner Truth, a Bondsman of Olden Time: With a History of Her Labors and Correspondence Drawn from Her "Book of Life."* New York: Oxford University Press, 1991.

hooks, bell, and Cornel West. *Breaking Bread: Insurgent Black Intellectual Life.* Boston, Mass.: South End Press, 1991.

Hopson, Darlene Powell and Derek S., *Different and Wonderful: Raising Black Children in a Race-Conscious Society.* New York: Prentice Hall, 1990.

Jewell, Terri L. *The Black Woman's Gumbo Ya-Ya: Quotations by Black Women.* Freedom, Calif.: Crossing Press, 1993.

Karenga, Maulana. *The African American Holiday of Kwanzaa: A Celebration of Family, Community, and Culture.* Los Angeles, Calif.: University of Sankore Press, 1988.

Lorde, Audre. *Sister Outsider: Essays and Speeches.* Trumansburg, N.Y.: Crossing Press, 1994.

Smith, Barbara. *Homegirls: A Black Feminist Anthology.* New York: Kitchen Table Press/Women of Color, 1983.

Van Sertima, Ivan. *Great Black Leaders, Ancient and Modern.* New Brunswick, N.J.: Transaction Books, 1988.

Welsing, Frances Cress. *The Isis (Yssis) Papers*. Chicago: Third World Press, 1991.

West, Cornel. *Race Matters*. Boston: Beacon Press, 1993.

Miscellaneous

Baldwin, James. *A Dialogue [by] James Baldwin [and] Nikki Giovanni*. Philadelphia, Pa.: Lippincott, 1973.

Butler, Octavia. *Kindred*. Garden City, N.Y.: Doubleday, 1979.

Evans, Mari. *Black Women Writers (1950–1980): A Critical Evaluation*. New York: Anchor/Doubleday, 1984.

Friday, Nancy. *My Mother, My Self: The Daughter's Search for Identity*. New York: Dell, 1977.

Gossett, Hattie. *Presenting Sister NoBlues*. Ithaca, N.Y.: Firebrand Press, 1988.

Matlins, Antoinette, Antonio Bonanno, and Jane Crystal. *Engagement and Wedding Rings: The Definitive Buying Guide for People in Love*. Vermont: Gemstone Press, 1990.

Morrison, Toni. *Playing in the Dark*. New York: Vintage, 1993.

Ruddick, Sara, and Pamela Daniels, eds. *Working It Out: Twenty-three Women Artists, Scientists, and Scholars Talk About Their Lives and Work*. New York: Pantheon, 1977.

Shange, Ntozake. *The Love Space Demands: A Continuing Saga*. New York: St. Martin's Press, 1991.

Walker, Alice, ed. *I Love Myself When I Am Laughing . . . and Then Again When I Am Looking Mean and Impressive: A Zora Neale Hurston Reader*. Old Westbury, N.Y.: Feminist Press, 1979.

Weinreb, Risa. *Frommer's Guide to Honeymoon Destinations*. New York: Prentice Hall, 1988.

Williams, Patricia J. *The Alchemy of Race and Rights*. Cambridge, Mass.: Harvard University Press, 1991.

BIBLIOGRAPHY

Aldridge, Delores P. *Focusing: Black Male-Female Relationships*. Chicago, Ill.: Third World Press, 1991.

Allen, Patrica. *Getting to "I Do."* New York: Morrow, 1994.

Anastasio, Janet, and Michelle Bevilacqua. *The Everything Wedding Vows Book*. Holbrook, Mass.: Bob Adams, 1994.

Artlip, Mary Ann, James A. Artlip, and Earl S. Saltzman. *The New American Family*. Lancaster, Pa.: Starburst Publishers, 1993.

Barreca, Regina. *Perfect Husbands (and Other Fairy Tales)*. New York: Anchor/Doubleday, 1993.

Bass, Ellen, and Laura Davis. *Beginning to Heal: A First Book for Survivors of Child Sexual Abuse*. New York: HarperCollins, 1993.

Bell, Alan P., and Martin Weinberg. *Homosexualities: A Study of Diversity Among Men and Women*. New York: Simon & Schuster, 1978.

Brook, Bryan. *Design Your Love Life: A Guide to Marriage and Relationships in the 90s*. New York: Walker, 1989.

Brothers, Joyce. *What Every Woman Ought to Know About Love and Marriage*. New York: Simon & Schuster, 1984.

Brown, Elaine. *A Taste of Power: A Black Woman's Story*. New York: Anchor/Doubleday, 1994.

Budge, Sir E. A. Wallis. *Egyptian Language*. New York: Dover, 1973.

Burr, Chandler. "Homosexuality and Biology," *The Atlantic*, March 1993.

Chandler, Joan. *Women Without Husbands: An Exploration of the Margins of Marriage*. New York: St. Martin's Press, 1991.

Chodorow, Nancy J. *Femininities, Masculinities, Sexualities: Freud and Beyond*. Lexington, Ky.: University Press of Kentucky, 1994.

Clark, Chris, and Sheila Rush. *How to Get Along with Black People: A Handbook for White Folks (And Some Black Folks Too)*. New York: The Third Press/Okpaku Publishing Co., 1971.

Cole, Harriette. *Jumping the Broom: The African American Wedding Planner*. New York: Holt, 1993.

Garber, Marjorie B. *Vice Versa: Bisexuality and the Eroticism of Everyday Life*. New York: Simon & Schuster, 1995.

Gawain, Shakti. *Creative Visualization*. San Rafael, Calif.: New World Library, 1978.

Gordon, Harley. *Remarriage Without Financial Risks: How to Do It Right the Next Time*. Boston, Mass.: Financial Planning Institute, 1992.

Hersey, Brook. *Bad Guys: Women's Tales from the Relationship Front*. New York: Bishop Books, 1994.

hooks, bell. *Talking Back: Thinking Feminist * Thinking Black*. Boston, Mass.: South End Press, 1989.

Hooper, Anne. *Anne Hooper's Pocket Sex Guide*. London: Dorling Kindersley, 1994.

Klein, Fritz. *The Bisexuality Option: A Concept of One Hundred Per Cent Intimacy*. Binghamton, N.Y.: Arbor House, 1978.

Leland, John. "Bisexuality Emerges as a New Sexual Identity." *Newsweek*, July 1995.

Major, Clarence. *Juba to Jive: A Dictionary of African American Slang*. New York: Penguin, 1994.

Maslin, Bonnie, and Yehuda Nir. *Not Quite Paradise: Making Marriage Work*. New York: Dolphin, 1987.

Metick, Sydney Barbara. *I Do: A Guide to Creating Your Own Unique Wedding Ceremony*. Berkeley, Calif.: Celestial Arts, 1992.

Moore, Rickie. *A Goddess in My Shoes: Seven Steps to Peace*. Atlanta, Ga.: Humanics New Age, 1988.

Moraga, Cherrie, and Gloria Anzaldua. *This Bridge Called My Back: Writings by Radical Women of Color*. New York: Kitchen Table/Women of Color Press, 1983.

Mullane, Deirdre. *Crossing the Danger Water: Three Hundred Years of African-American Writing*. New York: Anchor/Doubleday, 1993.

Oakley, Ann. *Subject Women: Where Women Stand Today—Politically, Socially, Emotionally*. New York: Pantheon, 1981.

Obudho, Constance. *Black Marriage and Family Therapy*. Westport, Conn.: Greenwood Press, 1983.

O'Neill, Nena and George. *Open Marriage: A New Lifestyle for Couples.* New York: Avon, 1972.

Peck, M. Scott. *The Road Less Traveled: A New Psychology of Love, Traditional Values, and Spiritual Growth.* New York, Simon & Schuster, 1978.

Pond, Mimi. *A Groom of One's Own and Other Bridal Accessories.* New York: Dutton, 1991.

Post, Elizabeth. *Emily Post on Second Weddings.* New York: HarperPerennial, 1991.

Putnam, James. *Life in Ancient Egypt.* London: Treasure Chests/Quarto Children's Books, 1994.

Roehrig, Catherine. *Fun with Hieroglyphs.* New York: The Metropolitan Museum of Art/Viking, 1990.

Rousseau, Mary, and Charles Gallagher. *Sexual Healing in Marriage.* Rockport, Mass.: Element Books, 1991.

Schlessinger, Laura. "The Cohabitation Trap," *Cosmopolitan,* March 1994.

Sevely, Josephine Lowndes. *Eve's Secrets.* New York: Random House, 1987.

Staple, Robert. *The World of Black Singles: Changing Patterns of Male/Female Relations.* Westport, Conn.: Greenwood Press, 1981.

Stoll, Clifford. *Silicon Snake Oil: Second Thoughts on the Information Highway.* New York: Doubleday, 1995.

Thorne, Tony. *The Dictionary of Contemporary Slang.* New York: Pantheon, 1990.

Vance, Carole S. *Pleasure and Danger: Exploring Female Sexuality.* Boston: Routledge & K. Paul, 1984.

White, Evelyn C. *The Black Women's Health Book: Speaking for Ourselves.* Seattle, Wash.: Seal Press, 1994.

Journal

Monique and Cassandra's 25 tips to Remember:

1. Get your act togethah, so when you finally do meet Mr. Right, he can't resist you.
2. Smile and say hello to every Black man you see.
3. Forgive old lovers and make peace with them.
4. Tell everyone you know that you're looking for a husband.
5. Go on as many blind dates as possible.
6. Date men who are not your "type"—you may be pleasantly surprised.
7. If you ask a man a series of questions within the first five minutes of meeting him, he'll tell you almost anything you want to know. After that he clams up and won't tell you a thing.
8. If you realize right away he is someone you don't like but does have an interesting job or hobby, he may have a friend who's perfect for you.
9. If he's available and you like him, don't hesitate to let him know it!
10. Dress conservatively. If you attract him with your body, how are you going to keep him with your mind?
11. Learn to listen.
12. Don't reveal all your charms right away.
13. If you've met and are dating a man you like, try to meet his family as soon as possible. You'd be surprised by how much you'll learn about him from just one visit with his folks.
14. Don't give unsolicited advice.
15. Once you've met him and you think he may be "The One," back off. Give him the space to pursue you.

16. Don't fall into the common trap of seeing only a man's "potential." Be realistic and see the man for who he is and where he is in his life right now.
17. Don't indulge an obsessive relationship.
18. Learn to compromise; it's one of the major challenges of marriage.
19. Don't let pride stand in the way.
20. Do not criticize or ridicule him.
21. Make sure he knows you love him by the care and attention you show him.
22. Tell him exactly what you'd like to do to him.
23. Don't be afraid to make him laugh or to laugh about things he says or does. This goes for when you're in bed as well!
24. Don't rule out men who are younger or older than you. Age is a matter of mind—if you don't mind, it doesn't matter!
25. Don't worry that there aren't loads of available men in your area. You only need one to marry!

(If you desire, this page may be cut out and placed in your wallet or daily planner for easy access!)